Living with Life-Threatening Illness

A Guide for Patients, Their
Families, and Caregivers

Kenneth J. Doka

Lexington Books

An Imprint of Macmillan, Inc.
New York

Maxwell Macmillan Canada
Toronto

Maxwell Macmillan International
New York · Oxford · Singapore · Sydney

Library of Congress Cataloging-in-Publication Data

Doka, Kenneth J.
    Living with life-threatening illness : a guide for patients, their families,
and caregivers / Kenneth J. Doka.
        p.   cm.
    Includes bibliographical references.
    ISBN 0-669-24227-6
    1. Catastrophic illness. 2. Catastrophic Illness—Patients-Family
relationships. 3. Terminal Care. 4. Caregivers.
I. Title
R726.5.5D65   1993
155.9'16—dc20   92—46186
                                                                            CIP

Lexington Books
An Imprint of Macmillan, Inc.
866 Third Avenue, New York, N.Y. 10022

Maxwell Macmillan Canada, Inc.
1200 Eglinton Avenue East
Suite 200
Don Mills, Ontario M3C 3N1

Macmillan, Inc. is part of the Maxwell Communication
Group of Companies.

Printed in the United States of America

printing number
1   2   3   4   5   6   7   8   9   10

To my Parents
Frank and Jay Doka
whose own struggles with life-threatening illness
taught me much about coping, caring, and courage

and to very special and longtime friends
Kathleen Dillon
Curt, Jill, Jake, and Amy Boyer
Eric and Cathy Schwarz
for their constant support and consistent love
in all the minor and major crises of life

Contents

Foreword

In a short story by Sherwood Anderson[*] entitled "Brother Death," there is a depiction of some events and relationships in the life of the Grey family. John and Louise Grey own a 1,200-acre cattle ranch in the blue grass country of the Rich Valley in southwestern Virginia. In addition to the parents, the family consists of five children: Don 18, Mary 14, Ted 11, Gladys 6, and Harry 2. Although the family is ostensibly well to do and happy, Anderson warns his readers that "people in your own family are likely at any moment to do strange, sometimes hurtful things to you. You have to watch them."

There are many levels and themes in this story. The most obvious is the sharp conflict that develops between the father, John, and the eldest son, Don, over the former's decision to cut down two large oak trees. These trees stand behind the house and are a favorite playground for the children. They represent humane and esthetic values, as well as the history of Louise's family which had planted them two generations earlier, against John's ambition and his desire to triumph over the past. In the conflict that develops, what begins almost as a casual thought on the part of John turns suddenly into stubborn determination when his decision is questioned, first by Louise and then by Don. When Don takes her side, Louise gives in to her husband in an effort to avoid serious conflict. But the matter has already come to involve the need of both father and son to assert themselves.

Another level of the story that is especially relevant here is the close bond that has developed between the two middle children, Mary and Ted. Ted has some kind of a heart condition, arising from a severe attack of diphtheria at the age of eight. As a result,

---

[*]Anderson, S. (1933). Brother death. In S. Anderson, *Death In the Woods and Other Stories* (pp. 271–298). New York: Liveright, Inc., Publishers.

"he was thin and not strong but curiously alive. The doctor said he might die at any moment, might just drop down dead."

Because he is living with a life-threatening condition, Ted's parents and older brother are overly protective toward him. They do not allow him to do many of the things that he wants to do. Only Mary realizes how hurtful this is to Ted and how he feels. Had Mary been able to articulate her thoughts, Anderson tells his readers, she might hae said: "If he is to have but a few years of life, they shall not spoil what he is to have. Why should they make him die, over and over, day after day?"

In her concern for Ted, Mary becomes like a soldier, standing guard over her brother. Everyone soon recognizes that the younger children have developed a special relationship, a world of their own in which Mary often acts as Ted's protector against others. Mary and Ted enjoy many good times together, but they are also quite serious. Once, when Mary criticizes her mother for stifling Ted's vitality, Anderson comments that "there was so much implied—even that Ted be allowed to die, quickly, suddenly, rather than that death, danger of sudden death, be brought again and again to his attention." From that day forward, things changed; Ted and Mary were granted new room to live as they needed.

In the conflict between John and Don over the oak trees, the lesson conveyed from father to son seems to be that "something in you must die before you can possess and command." The father's decision prevailed and Don's submission is a kind of "little death." A year or two later, Ted dies quietly in his bed during the night, but in the meantime he is able to live with a curious sense of freedom and without further protests from his parents. In short, says Anderson, Ted "would never have to face the more subtle and terrible death that had come to his older brother."

In the book that follows, Kenneth Doka draws attention to the many elements involved in living with a life-threatening illness. The great strength of this book is the breadth of its vision and the depth of its analysis. Doka recognizes clearly that living and coping with a life-threatening illness is not just a matter of feelings. Instead, he emphasizes the many efforts individuals exert in order to try and manage the challenges that arise from life-threatening illness. This includes efforts addressed to the physical, psychological, social, and spiritual dimensions of such challenges.

Further, Doka rightly recognizes that there are different challenges to face at different points in the journey that is involved in coping with a life-threatening illness. An illness of this sort is not simply a single, unified entity. It presents itself in quite different ways at different points in its progression. In this book, Doka does readers the very great service of identifying and describing key points that are associated with life-threatening illness: before diagnosis; at the time of diagnosis; during the lengthy chronic phase that increasingly characterizes the sorts of degenerative diseases that are life-threatening in contemporary society; at the point of recovery, if that is what happens; and at or near the point of death, if that is the eventual outcome.

Another feature of Doka's analysis is that it is not just confined to the ill person. The group of those who are coping with a life-threatening illness includes the ill person, his or her "family" (however its members may be defined), and those who provide care to that person (family members, friends, professionals, and volunteers alike). Coping is an activity of individual persons, but it is not merely a matter for isolated individuals. Each individual copes with his or her own challenges, as well as with the needs and behaviors of others in the human coping network.

In short, coping is different at different points in the illness trajectory, at different points in the life cycle, and for different individuals who are drawn into involvement with a life-threatening illness. The reason for this is that coping processes are the constantly changing ways in which living human beings attempt to manage stressful challenges. Such challenges arise from illness, dying, personal needs, and interpersonal relationships. Coping with such challenges is an activity of living persons and interdependent human beings. If these individuals were not alive, there would be no reason to expend energy in actively listening to and appreciating the evolving kaleidoscope of ways in which each person is living out his or her involvements with life-threatening illness.

Coping involves effort. Efforts can be described in terms of tasks. Every living individual chooses to exert his or her efforts in his or her own ways. That is, in coping each person undertakes tasks (or sets them aside) at a time, pace and way of his or her own choosing. *Living with Life-Threatening Illness* offers a rich description of ways in which human beings are both alike and different in coping with the hazards of life and death. Even though none of us can control the whole of a life-threatening illness, Doka's analysis demonstrates that there are many ways in which we can take charge or attempt to manage many aspects of the challenges it presents. In so doing, we have an opportunity to improve quality in living, even when that living is conducted in very difficult circumstances. In so doing, the pressures of life-threatening illness disclose the preciousness of life itself and the indomitable vitality of the human spirit.

Those who read this book owe a debt of gratitude to its author for helping us to achieve a better understanding and appreciation of ourselves and of our fellow human beings who are engaged in living and coping with life-threatening illness.

Charles A. Corr
Southern Illinois University
at Edwardsville

Introduction

- A thirty-six-year-old mother of four learns that the tingling in her arm has been diagnosed as multiple sclerosis.
- A sixty-four-year-old man, experiencing chest pains, is told he is having a heart attack.
- The parents of a two-year-old boy sit anxiously in a doctor's office, waiting to learn why their son has experienced continuous fevers and bruises so easily.
- A twenty-eight-year-old architect finds that he is HIV positive.
- During a routine examination a sixty-nine-year-old man is informed that he has a spot on his lung.
- Parents of a two month old are told that their son has cystic fibrosis.
- A forty-one-year-old physician finds a lump in her breast.

In all these cases individuals and their families are facing a moment of crisis, a terrible trial, a frightening encounter with mortality. Each must decide upon a course of action, when to seek medical help, how to choose the best treatment. The experiences of all these people may be very different. Some may find that their worst fears are not realized. The lump may turn out to be merely a cyst, the spot on the lung may be benign. Some may undergo surgery or chemotherapy and eventually recover, but be forever changed by the experience of illness. Others may struggle with chronic illness. And still others may face impending death.

The experience of life-threatening illness is one of the most difficult situations that individuals and their families ever have to face. From the first mounting suspicions about dangerous symptoms through the crisis of diagnosis and long periods of chronic illness, whether the result is recovery or death, any encounter with life-threatening illness leaves an indelible mark on ill individuals, their families, and even the people who care for them.

This book is meant to be a guide for anyone caught in the struggle with life-threatening illness: individuals, their families, or caregivers. Its very title, *Living with Life-Threatening Illness,* recognizes the medical revolution that has so radically changed the experience of illness. Years ago to be diagnosed with any of a number of "fatal" diseases was to receive a virtual death sentence. A person with such a serious disease could expect to live but a short time; indeed, he or she might never leave the hospital.

Often now the experience of serious illness is dramatically different. Individuals can live a long time with life-threatening illness. Some—increasingly greater numbers each year—will recover. Most will leave hospitals even as they continue treatment. Many will resume their former lives, going back to work or to school even as they continue to struggle with disease. Only at the very end of this process, often years after the initial diagnosis, will some finally reach the terminal phase of their illness. Living with life-threatening illness is the theme of this book as it describes the particular challenges that individuals, families, and caregivers face at varying points during serious illness.

Every book has its own biography. This book really arises from two sources. For the past twenty years I have taught courses on dying and death. In that teaching, particularly in a graduate seminar for nurses and other caregivers, I began to incorporate additional material that reflected the changed reality of illness, dying, and death that has occurred since the 1969 publication of Kubler-Ross's epochal *On Death and Dying*. My classes began to consider issues related to the diagnosis of illness such as decisions about when to seek medical help or to take such diagnostic tests as the HIV test. We also started to address issues associated with the problem of living with chronic illness. In short, we began to look at the dying process in the larger context of life-threatening illness. We studied the writings of E. Mansell Pattison (1969, 1978) and Avery Weisman (1980), two pioneering clinical researchers who emphasized the idea that life-threatening illness is a long process, best viewed as series of phases, each with its own unique issues and problems. This book owes a heavy debt to their insights as well as to the work of many writers, researchers, and clinicians who are mentioned in the references. The bibliography lists all the sources that I have found helpful while writing this book, but I wish to acknowledge my special debts to the work of Corr (1991), Kalish (1985), Moos (1977, 1984), Rando (1984), and Strauss (1975).

My father's bout with cancer also helped me to organize my own thoughts about the ways we look at life-threatening illness. It reminded me of the uncertainty that we often face as we struggle with illness. Diagnosis can be an uncertain process, a roller coaster of good and bad news. Prognosis is rarely certain and time frames can only be expressed as probabilities. The struggle is draining, not just for the ill individuals, but for their families and their caregivers. It taught me two additional lessons. First, that people do recover, as did my father, but that even in recovery the experience leaves residual effects. Second, it reminded me that this work draws from a second critial source, the experiences and responses that so many people have shared with me throughout these past twenty years. While their names are not listed in any of the references, they too have taught me much about living with life-threatening illness.

Throughout my career I have resisted the term "patient." I have always found the term "patient" to be inaccurate because it suggests that the ill individual is totally passive. For much of the struggle with life-threatening illness, individuals are rarely patients in the sense that they are spending much of their time in hospitals or physician's offices. The root of the word *patient* actually means "someone being acted upon." That idea too was objectionable, for I have always stressed that individuals respond best to life-threatening illness when they are active participants in their own treatment.

One colleague, struggling herself with life-threatening illness, likes to call herself a "protagonist." Drawn from Greek drama, the term "protagonist" refers to the central character around which all action revolves. It is the protagonist who sets the pace and direction for the ensuing drama. I have often felt that her perception of her role, her demand to be the pivotal character in her own life struggle, is the key factor in her long survival. I hope we come to the time soon when all persons with life-threatening illness will define themselves as protagonists.

Given my strong negative feelings about the word *patient*, I tried to avoid its use as much as possible in this book. At times, though, "patient" seemed the best and most clear way to refer to individuals with an illness. Yet, "patient" is clearly familiar, and after much thought, it seemed the most suitable term to use in the subtitle. Also, in certain contexts such as a hospital, other terms such as "persons with illness," "victims," or "clients" seemed awkward, unclear, artificial, and sometimes even stigmatizing.

I deliberately chose to use the term "life-threatening illness" rather than terms such as "catastrophic illness," "fatal illness," or "terminal illness." A life-threatening illness is any illness that endangers life or that has significant risk of death. The term "catastrophic illness" seemed to overemphasize the crisis nature of the illness. Though there are times of crisis, and a diagnosis can truly be catastrophic, the term "catastrophic illness" tends to underemphasize the reality that many people strive to maintain a normal life even when faced with impending death. In this book people are only referred to as "dying" when they are in the final, terminal phase of life-threatening illness. In the terminal phase the illness has progressed to such a point that recovery or remission is highly improbable, health has declined, and death is likely to occur within a specific time frame.

One of the central lessons I have learned is that every experience of life-threatening illness is distinct, and individual responses are therefore very different. Chapters 1 and 2 explore and emphasize that individuality. People respond to life-threatening illness in a variety of ways. A wise instructor once told me that he could predict the way I would die. When I asked "How?," he answered, "The same way you respond to any life crisis." Chapter 1 considers the range of responses to life-threatening illness that individuals, their families, and other caregivers may experience.

Responses to illness are affected by many factors. No two experiences of illness are alike. Each disease creates its own special issues and particular problems. Nor is coping with a disease an isolated process. Rather, it is a part of the continuing process of life, influenced by all the developmental, psychological, and social factors that influence response to any life crisis. These factors are described in Chapter 2.

Chapters 3 through 7 describe particular issues that arise at different points during the experience of life-threatening illness. Underlying this book is a perspective or model that views life-threatening illness as a series of phases, each with its particular challenges or tasks (see the model).

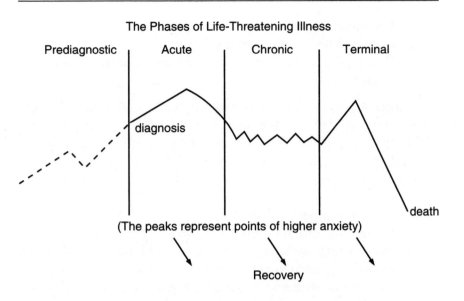

The Phases of Life-Threatening Illness

Corr (1991) indicates that these challenges include physical ones (for example, the physical changes caused by disease and treatment), psychological ones (for example, maintaining a sense of psychological comfort in the face of disease), social ones (for example, negotiating relationships and roles changed by the fact of illness), and spiritual ones (for example, finding meaning and value in the midst of illness). All dimensions of our life are affected by an encounter with illness and death.

Chapters 3 through 7 describe those tasks and offer suggestions for coping. I use the term "task" quite deliberately. As Corr (1991) reminds us, "task" does not imply any order or sequence. Each task simply refers to challenges posed for many people at different points in life-threatening illness. The use of this term also reinforces a personal sense of freedom. Just as any individual can decide on any day that he or she will choose to do or not to do particular chores, so individuals struggling with life-threatening illness can also choose to confront or not to confront particular challenges or tasks presented by the illness. These tasks can be outlined in the following way:

A *Prediagnostic phase,* discussed in Chapter 3, often precedes diagnosis. Here, someone recognizes symptoms or risk factors that make him or her prone to illness. That person now needs to select strategies to cope with this threat. The tasks here include:

1. Recognizing possible danger or risk.
2. Coping with anxiety and uncertainty
3. Developing and following through on a health-seeking strategy.

Chapter 4 considers the *Acute phase* that centers around the crisis of diagnosis. At this point an individual is faced with a diagnosis of life-threatening illness and must make a series of decisions—medical, psychological, interpersonal, and so on—about how, at least initially, to cope with this crisis. Here the tasks include:

1. Understanding the disease
2. Examining and maximizing health and life-style
3. Maximizing one's coping strengths and limiting weaknesses
4. Examining internal and external resources and liabilities
5. Developing strategies to deal with issues created by disease (disclosure, coping with professionals, treatment options, life contingencies)
6. Exploring the effect of illness on one's sense of self and relationships with others
7. Ventilating feelings and fears
8. Integrating the present reality of the diagnosis with one's past life and future plans.

Chapter 5 describes the *Chronic phase*. During this period an individual is struggling with the disease and its treatment. Many people in this phase may be attempting, with varying degrees of success, to live a reasonably normal life within the confines of the disease. Often this period is puncutated by a series of illness-related crises. Tasks in this phase (see Lubkin 1986; Strauss 1975) include:

1. Managing symptoms and side effects
2. Carrying out health regimens
3. Preventing and managing health crises
4. Managing stress and examining coping
5. Maximizing social support and minimizing social isolation
6. Normalizing life in the face of disease
7. Dealing with financial concerns
8. Preserving self-concept

9. Redefining relationships with others throughout the course of disease
10. Ventilating feelings and fears
11. Finding meaning in suffering, chronicity, uncertainty, and decline.

In many cases people will not experience all of these phases. Sometimes in the acute or chronic phase, or even rarely in the terminal phase, a person may experience recovery. This *Recovery phase* is described in Chapter 6. Even here, however, people may have to cope with certain tasks such as:

1. Dealing with psychological, social, physical, spiritual, and financial aftereffects of illness
2. Coping with fears and anxieties about recurrence
3. Examining life and life-style issues and reconstructing one's life
4. Redefining relationships with caregivers.

Chapter 7 reviews the *Terminal phase*. This describes the situation in which the disease has progressed to a point where death is inevitable. Death is no longer merely *possible*; now it is *likely*. Death has become the individual's and family's central crisis. Tasks (see Rando 1984; Kalish 1985) here include:

1. Dealing with symptoms, discomfort, pain, and incapacitation
2. Managing health procedures and institutional procedures
3. Managing stress and examining coping
4. Dealing effectively with caregivers
5. Preparing for death and saying good-bye
6. Preserving self-concept
7. Preserving appropriate relationships with family and friends
8. Ventilating feelings and fears
9. Finding meaning in life and death.

To summarize, this model holds that in any experience with life-threatening illness one is faced with four major tasks:

1. Responding to the physical fact of disease
2. Taking steps to cope with the reality of disease
3. Preserving self-concept and relationships with others in the face of disease

4. Dealing with the affective and existential/spiritual issues created or reactivated by the disease.

At each phase of the illness, these basic tasks may raise different issues, concerns, and challenges (see Table 1).

It is important to remember that while this model can be useful, at best it offers a *general* description of a complicated and highly *individual* process. Not every individual will experience the situations and reactions I describe here. Nor will every life-threatening illness proceed methodically or precisely through these phases. In many cases an individual will seek medical treatment, fearing the worst, and happily find that the symptom is minor and the condition itself easily treated. Even a diagnosis of life-threatening illness can result in successful surgeries or other interventions that minimize or eliminate any further risk. In many illnesses, such as multiple sclerosis, a chronic phase can last indefinitely, while with other illnesss declines into a terminal phase will immmediately follow diagnosis.

There is another limitation to this model. We need to remember that life-threatening illness is only part of life. Throughout the time of the illness, at whatever phase, individuals continue to meet many needs and to cope with all the issues and problems that they had prior to the diagnosis. The experience of illness may affect the perception of these needs and issues as well as ways of coping. These earlier needs and issues, however, continue throughout the illness. While this model emphasizes the experience of the illness, living with life-threatening illness recognizes that all the previous challenges of life—dealing with family and friends, coping with work and finances, even keeping up with the demands of a home or apartment—remain an ongoing part of that larger struggle.

Life-threatening illness is inevitably a family illness, for the life of everyone with the family is changed when one member of a family experiences disease. Chapter 8 considers the ways in which families may be affected by illness. It also offers suggestions for helping families to cope with the illness of a family member.

Chapter 9 applies this general discussion to the special needs of specific populations such as children, the developmentally disabled, and the elderly, as well as those of different cultures. Chapter 10, specifically intended for health professionals and other

TABLE I

Tasks in Life-Threatening Illness

Prediagnostic Phase	Acute Phase	Chronic Phase	Terminal Phase
1. Responding to the physical fact of disease 2. Taking steps to cope with the reality of disease	1. Understanding the disease 2. Maximizing health and lifestyle 3. Maximizing one's coping strengths and limiting weaknesses 4. Developing strategies to deal with the issues created by the disease	1. Managing symptoms and side effects 2. Carrying out health regimens 3. Preventing and managing health crisis 4. Managing stress and examining coping 5. Maximizing social support and minimizing isolation 6. Normalizing life in the face of the disease 7. Dealing with financial concerns	1. Dealing with symptoms, discomfort, pain, and incapacitation 2. Managing health procedures and institutional stress 3. Managing stress and examining coping 4. Dealing effectively with caregivers 5. Preparing for death and saying goodbye
3. Preserving self concept and relationships with others in the face of disease 4. Dealing with affective and existential/spiritual issues created or reactivated by the disease	5. Exploring the effect of the diagnosis on a sense of self and others 6. Ventilating feelings and fears 7. Incorporating the present reality of diagnosis into one's sense of past and future	8. Preserving self concept 9. Redefining relationships with others throughout the course of the disease 10. Ventilating feelings and fears 11. Finding meaning in suffering, chronicity, uncertainty and decline	6. Preserving self concept 7. Preserving appropriate relationships with family and friends 8. Ventilating feelings and fears 9. Finding meaning in life and death

caregivers, stresses the special roles that they may have in assisting individuals and families who are coping with life-threatening illness. It also recognizes the special sense of loss that is part of that role.

A number of years ago one of my students, soon after taking my dying and death course, found that her brother, with whom she was very close, had cancer. She nursed him, helped her parents, and struggled with her own emotions. One day she came to class to talk about her experiences in coping with his illness and subsequent death. Someone asked her if the course had helped. She answered, "It didn't change my feelings or the situations and crises we faced. It did make them more understandable." That really expresses the goal of this book: to make the struggle with life-threatening illness a little more understandable, and perhaps less lonely and frightening.

Responses to Life-Threatening Illness

Rob and John share a room in a hospital. Both are dying of cancer. Beyond their illness they have little in common. Rob is a forty-nine-year-old African-American who works as a bank manager. Always taught to be polite, he is a model of graciousness to the staff. Brought up in a strict Pentecostal faith, he is consumed by a sense of guilt that this illness is the result of some yet-undiscovered sin. John is a sixty-seven-year-old retired steamfitter. Always a brawler with a fearsome temper, he is still angry, constantly lashing out at family and staff.

These two men illustrate an important point. Each of us will die much as we live. The ways by which one currently responds to everyday crises often give clues as to how one will respond to the crisis of illness or death. Thus it is useful to explore the ways one has responded to crisis in the past. Often we can be expected to show similar reactions now.

In 1969 Elizabeth Kubler-Ross, in her now-famous *On Death and Dying*, described five common responses to a crisis of dying: denial, anger, bargaining, depression, and acceptance. Unfortunately, many readers mistakenly believed that everyone who was dying responded in those same five ways and in that order, something Kubler-Ross never meant to say. Many people began to use Kubler-Ross's stages as a therapeutic model, trying to move people into acceptance because they believed that to be the most desired state.

Many researchers and clinicians now emphasize the idea that each individual has his or her own vision of what is an appropriate death. To some it may mean peacefully accepting death. To others it may mean fighting death bitterly to the end. Still others might choose to die quickly or opt for heavy sedation. *Each* person has his or her own definition of a "good death."

Researchers and clinicians also stress that the ways we respond and react to the crisis of death are also highly individual and varied. Shneidman (1978), a pioneer in death studies, has characterized dying persons as exhibiting a "hive of affect." By that, Shneidman meant that dying persons can rarely be characterized in terms of a single emotional response such as "anger" at any given point in the illness. Rather, they may experience a range of many—sometimes contradictory—emotions simultaneously. Think, for example, of a life crisis as minor as an adolescent who has not returned at curfew. Parents experiencing this minor crisis may be experiencing anger, guilt, anxiety, disappointment, and sadness, all at the same time. Responses to life-threatening illness are not only experienced on the emotional level but on physical, behavioral, cognitive, and even spiritual levels as well. This chapter describes the many types of responses that individuals can have as they cope with personal or familial crises of life-threatening illness and death.

Physical Responses

Physical Manifestations of Stress

The diagnosis of life-threatening illness is an extraordinarily stressful event. This intense crisis begins with the diagnosis itself. While the sense of crisis may recede during the chronic phase, new stressors including treatment, accommodating the demands of life as the illness continues, and often a continued uncertainty, will arise. Stress itself can become chronic at this time. In the terminal phase dying itself is an unresolvable crisis. This too creates acute stress.

Many individuals will manifest this continuing stress physically. The range of physical reactions to stress can include insomnia, headaches, dizziness, fatigue, nausea, tingling sensations, and a variety of other physical ills. One should alert one's physician if experiencing any of these reactions, for physical responses, particularly changes in eating and sleeping patterns, may also result from the effects of the disease and treatments.

Preoccupation with Health

In life-threatening illness many people begin to shift their focus inward. A natural result of the trauma of diagnosis is that one can become extremely aware of and sensitive to one's body. Given this heightened anxiety and a preoccupation with oneself, minor symptoms and sensations, once ignored or quickly dismissed, may become the focus of considerable attention and concern. It is also normal during serious illness to become particularly sensitive to certain physical reactions that one fears may indicate particular dangers, such as relapse, metastasis, or reoccurrence. For example, one woman recovering from breast cancer became extremely concerned about back pain. Investigation revealed that her concern was instigated by a dying woman she had met in the hospital who described such pain as the first symptom that her breast cancer had metastasized. This preoccupation with health can affect anyone who is ill; indeed, a concern with health is heightened whenever one faces illness, even the illness of another. Illness tends to remind one of one's own vulnerability. One takes chest pains much more seriuosly when a friend has had a heart attack.

Again, it is important to report any symptoms to a physician. This is critical in order for the physician to monitor the illness and treatment. When someone you love is seriously ill, you should monitor your own health. Regular physical examinations with a physician who is aware of your situation may help you realize the ways in which the stress of another's illness may be affecting one's own health. Healthy life-style practices such as good nutrition, regular exercise, adequate rest and relaxation, and effective stress management are all especially important in stressful times.

Pain and Suffering

Pain is not only a physical manifestation of illness, one that may be evident in different degrees throughout the phases of illness. Pain may also be seen as a response to life-threatening illness. One must distinguish between *"pain,"* which is a perception of physical sensations, and *"suffering,"* which is an emotional response to that physical perception. The distinction allows us to understand that life-threatening illness not only causes pain, it generates suffering. Pain is a physical fact of illness; suffering is how one responds to the fact of illness.

Pain and suffering may be experienced on many levels. First, there is the physical pain which can be acute and intense or chronic. Again, as with any physical reaction, it is important to report pain to a physician. In some cases pain can be an important tool to assist the physician in diagnosis or in monitoring treatment. One should also discuss ways that pain can be alleviated or controlled.

Beyond the physical, there are other forms of pain and suffering as well. Pain and suffering may be experienced on psychological, social, spiritual, sexual, and financial levels. Pain and suffering can be intensely felt. For many persons with life-threatening illness the reality of pain becomes the critical issue. Pain and suffering can become their primary focus, and in some cases the sole topic of conversation.

Cognitive Responses

Shock

Often one's initial response to life-threatening illness is a profound sense of shock. Just as humans will respond to severe physical trauma by going into shock, a person can respond to the psychological trauma of a serious diagnosis with a similar reaction. This may be evident in high levels of stress, as well as confusion, disorientation, and numbness.

Denial

One of the most common and complex responses to life-threatening illness is denial. However as Weisman (1972) indicates, there are a number of different levels of denial. For example, Weisman defines "first-order denial" as a denial of the facts. Here one denies the symptoms of the illness: "This is not really a lump or, if it is, it is a result of an earlier injury." This form of denial often occurs in the prediagnostic phase where it may delay seeking medical help. "Second"- and "third-order denial" are more common in the later phases of illness. In "second-order denial" one admits the symptoms and diagnosis but refuses to acknowledge the implications of that diagnosis. One often focuses on each symptom, crisis, or event as an isolated item. A person with cancer, for example, may focus on an impending operation, giving little attention to the long-term implications of the disease. "Third-order denial" occurs when one recognizes an incurable disease but still views the illness as indefinitely prolonged. In other words, one denies the possibility of death. For example, in one case a thirty-year-old person with AIDS shared his diagnosis with a counselor, but then indicated that he expected to live to be seventy, the average age when males in his family died.

Denial is also made more complex by the fact that what seems like denial can, in fact, be many other things. One of the key issues of life-threatening illness, especially in its early phases, is managing information about that illness. One needs to make decisions about who to tell, when to share that information, and what to say about the disease. Work, promotions, relationships, even self-esteem may be affected by these decisions. It is not unusual to guard this information carefully, perhaps by emphasizing the most optimistic scenarios or even by using evasion and deception. These (mis)communciations may shed little light on the person's own awareness of illness. Also, one can consciously choose to suppress the fact of illness, remaining aware of the disease and its implications but concentrating on less-traumatic issues.

There may be a very thin line between public acknowledgment and private awareness of illness. Weisman (1972) uses the phrase "middle knowledge" to express the complex reality of awareness and denial. Dying people may drift in and out of awareness of death. At some points they may acknowledge, selectively to given individuals, the seriousness of their illness, while at other times they may seemingly ignore such issues.

Denial in the early phases of illness is not only common but also understandable. Many serious life-threatening illnesses such as HIV infection or chronic lymphocytic leukemia, are asymptomatic in the early stages. Other life-threatening diseases typically include extended periods of remission. For many life-threatening diseases prognosis is uncertain. It is certainly natural to avoid the possible implications of threatened survival.

Denial may also be functional. It is not always negative. Sometimes it helps people adjust to illness. A degree of denial allows us to continue to plan for the future, maintain social relationships, and even participate in treatment. After all, it makes little sense to submit to painful treatment if there is no possibility of ultimate beneficial effect. Denial may be adaptive when recognition will not alter the situation. It may be very useful early in the illness as a way of mitigating the threat. And there is even some tentative research (Weisman and Worden 1975) that indicates denial is associated with longer survival. In all of these circumstances, denial may have a useful role to play and should not be condemned by outsiders.

Denial should only be considered a problem when it constitutes a threat to the health of a person or others. For example, a person who denies the seriousness of his illness or who maintains an irrational delusion of health so that it affects participation in or adherence to treatment may need to be questioned. This problem often occurs during periods of remission when the ill person, encouraged by recovered health, denies an initially accepted diagnosis. Signs of such denial may be evidenced by relaxed adherence to treatment or even its total suspension. In one case a man who had suffered from heart failure experienced a significant gain in health after initial treatment. He then became convinced that the original diagnosis was a mistake, a result of mixed test results, and he stopped taking his medication and visiting the outpatient clinic. The unfortunate result was that his health rapidly deteriorated.

Similarly, a caregiver may need to confront a person who endangers the health of others, such as a person who is HIV positive but who denies infection and continues to participate in behaviors that have a high risk of transmitting the virus to others. Here, counterproductive denial jeopardizes the welfare of others. In other cases, denial should be recognized for what it is, a psychological defense that buffers an individual from encountering a severe psychological threat in the circumstances that the person may be unable to handle.

It is always valuable to allow the person to honestly explore, at his or her own pace, any concerns that may develop. Given the reality of "middle knowledge," people will at times address issues of illness, physical deterioration, or dying and at other moments they will entertain hopes for eventual recovery. But in an understanding and accepting context, the person may, at times, choose to let down the defense of denial.

Egocentricity and Constriction of Interests

At the time of diagnosis one may turn inward. One can become egocentric, severely limiting all outside interests. There are many reasons for this. Physiological factors focus attention on bodily sensations: one becomes tuned into one's own body during illness. Psychologically, the crisis of diagnosis centers all attention on the illness, the source of the stress. In addition, interactions with others may be limited by hospitalization, the attention of family and friends, and the attempt to spare them further stress or to exempt them from role responsibilities. Even family members caught in the crisis may experience that same sense of egocentricity.

Generally, as one moves from the crisis of the diagnostic phase into the chronic phase, egocentricity tends to diminish. Here hope for continued existence may strongly reemerge. In addition, the challenges, diversion, and stimulation of resumed roles tends to refocus attention outward. Both the ill person and other family members have gone back to work or school and family life, and a degree of normalcy returns. In many cases, though, some egocentricity and constriction of interests may still be observed during the chronic phase. Treatment and symptoms are constant reminders of disease. Fears of deterioration, relapse, or reoccurrence place constraints on any future planning. The fact of illness, the demands of treatment, lessened energy levels, and even decisions on priorities may diminish or end involvement in certain activities and roles.

As health begins to deteriorate, especially in the terminal phase, egocentricity and constriction of interests are likely to reemerge. Often, disengagement of the dying individual from others is a clear sign of impending death. The dying person seems to withdraw from others, and lacks interest in any outside needs. This disengagement may be a manifestation of underlying depression and grief, a psychological reaction to unresolvable crisis, a response to the withdrawal of others, or a reflective struggle as the person focuses attention on inward spiritual needs.

Bargaining

Bargaining too has been identified as a common response to a life-threatening illness. Bargaining is a feeling that by omitting or committing certain actions one can avoid or forestall further illness or death. It is often expressed through explicit or implicit "deals" with some figure of authority. For example, bargaining may revolve around life-style and adherence issues. One may promise to amend certain life-style practices that contributed to the illness or may agree to accept medical treatment.

One may exhibit an almost magical thinking about adherence to the medical regimen. "If only I watch my diet, take my medication, and do everything I am told, I will achieve continued remission or cure." Sometimes this can have an initial positive aspect in encouraging adherence to the medical regimen, but later in the course of the disease the impact can be negative when the individual feels disenchantment and discouragement as the illness proceeds. Thus it is important for caregivers to provide hopeful yet realistic messages about what adherence to the medical regimen is likely to achieve.

Sometimes we may perceive that a change in life-style will ensure health. A gay man with AIDS once stated, "I became sick because I engaged in promiscuous and unsafe sex. If I stop doing what made me sick, I will stay well." A person with heart disease promised God he would attend church regularly if the operation was successful. The turning toward religion that has often been observed in persons diagnosed with life-threatening illness may be, at least in part, a manifestation of the "bargaining" response to illness.

The nature of bargains often strongly reflects the person's experience of illness. Early on in the illness bargains may emphasize cures or significant remission. Later, as the individual begins to experience deterioration, bargains may focus on living to enjoy certain significant events or milestones (such as birthdays, anniversaries, a daughter's wedding, and so on), living pain-free, or even on an afterlife.

Bargaining can have both constructive and destructive aspects. In some cases it can facilitate life-enhancing behaviors. In others, however, it can lead to feelings that may inhibit adaptation. For example, in one case a twenty-five-year-old male homosexual feared HIV infection. He promised that if the tests proved negative he would give up dangerous sexual practices, a promise he kept during the interim between taking the test and receiving the results. When the results were positive he felt a strong sense of betrayal and deep feelings of pessimism and anger. He then returned to risky sexual behavior.

In the chronic phase of illness such bargains may continue to encourage adherence. Individuals may believe that as long as they participate in treatment that will forestall continued decline. However, should deterioration continue, individuals may feel discouraged and angry that the "bargain" was not kept, losing motivation for adherence to treatment.

Changes in Body Image and Self-Esteem

Every culture values its own image of physical vitality and attractiveness. The combination of disease and treatment can cause effects that undermine a person's sense of physical attractiveness, thereby impairing body image. Since body image is so interwoven with sexuality, gender identity, self-concept, and self-esteem, the effects on body image can be highly significant.

Goffman (1963), in his book *Stigma*, described the impacts of stigma or impaired body image on self-concept. To Goffman, stigma creates a discrepancy between actual and virtual social identity; that is, there is a difference between the way someone would like to view himself or herself and the way others perceive him or her. Often this stigma affects both interaction and identity. The following cases illustrates the stigma that chronic illness creates.

> *Barbara is an attractive forty-nine-year-old woman with cancer. She had an operation that left scarring on her abdomen. She also received chemotherapy that sometimes made her appear bloated. Though a very attractive woman, she is very sensitive about the scars on her body, even though they are relatively minor. She feels much less attractive since surgery. A divorcee, involved in a serious relationship with a man, she has not been able to have sex since her first surgery. She worries that eventually her boyfriend will leave her and she will live on as a "lonely old, ugly woman."*
>
> *Tommy, a twelve year old with cancer, has a series of surgical scars on his chest. Once athletic and involved on many teams he now avoids swimming or basketball. He even hates to change for gym since he is reluctant to take off his shirt in*

the locker-room. He tends to be far more withdrawn and less social than he was prior to the surgery.

Changes in body image caused by disease and treatment can affect other aspects of identity and self-esteem. It is important to note that body image has a subjective reality. One's body image may plummet even when objective changes seem only minor.

Near-Death Experiences

Since the publication of Moody's *Life after Life* in 1975, there has been considerable interest in "near-death experiences" or "altered consciousness experiences." As Moody describes it, persons near death often experience a common sequence of events in which they experience their body moving through a dark tunnel, glimpsing the spirits of others who have died. To Moody these experiences were warm and positive and often left survivors with a lessened fear of death.

Near-death experiences are not uncommon in life-threatening illness. But they do not seem to be universal or uniform. Nor are they always comforting and positive. Some researchers (Kastenbaum, 1979) have found that many individuals have experienced frightening episodes involving terrifying images. Further, such experiences may have many possible explanations. Some people (eg. Moody, 1975) feel they may represent proof of an afterlife, while others (Kastenbaum, 1979) hold that they may be a reaction to drugs or internal chemical changes.

The key issue is how the individual who has this experience interprets it, and whether he or she finds it comforting. Caregivers should ask individuals if they have had any such experiences and then allow them to recount and interpret that experience.

Dreams and Sleep Disturbances

During a life-threatening illness sleep disturbances are common. Stress and uncertainty may lead to bouts of insomnia. An individual may be troubled by dreams that reflect preoperative anxieties, anxieties associated with illness or treatment, or fears of death. One man facing amputation dreamt he was in a butcher shop with limbs and body parts hanging from meat hooks. In another case a newly diagnosed MS patient dreamt she was invisible as she frantically tried to receive help from family and friends, thereby reflecting her fears of abandonment and death.

Dreams may sometimes reflect spiritual anxieties, especially during the acute and terminal phase. For example, one woman who was facing surgery was deeply troubled by her decision to bring up her children in a faith different from the one in which she had been raised. She began to have recurrent dreams in which she saw a poker table covered with pennies. (Penny poker was her major form of recreation.) Each penny had a different face. A large finger that she assumed was the hand of God was separating the pennies into different piles. She would always wake up when the finger was placed upon her face.

Dreams do not always have to be fearful. One adolescent, soon after his diagnosis of a brain tumor, had a dream about a "peaceful warrior." This warrior was able to surmount numerous obstacles to resolve his quest and prove his manhood. The dream became a metaphor, providing inner strength for the youth's struggle with his illness. Dreams, then, are an effective way to reflect upon a person's underlying concern. Again, caregivers do well to ask people what they have dreamed, and to encourage them to explore and interpret these dreams.

Existential Plight, Reassessment of Life, and Mortality

Confronting life-threatening illness often leads to an intensified awareness of one's own mortality. Facing death often causes both the individual and family members to review and make sense of their past lives, and to assess the present and future as well. One may reassess one's values, beliefs, and priorities. This struggle can sometimes intensify feelings of anger, anxiety, and guilt. An individual may feel bitter or guilty about missed opportunities, prior choices, or unfinished business. He may ponder what he has done to deserve this disease. She may even fall into despair over the meaning of her own existence.

There may be positive aspects as well. Often an individual will make decisions that will enhance the quality of life. It is not unusual for persons who experience life-threatening illness to speak of the illness as a turning point in their lives; because of their illness they reordered their priorities, thereby enriching the quality of whatever time remains. Some people are able to construct systems of thought that allow them to integrate and interpret their experience of illness in ways that enhance self-esteem. One man struggling with a crippling disease found comfort in the fact that it caused him to think more about his family. He was able to reinterpret the time he was forced to stay at home as an opportunity to reconnect with his children. The knowledge of mortality may give present life new vitality, even turning mundane tasks into pleasurable achievements.

Cognitive Impairments and Psychiatric Disturbances

The tremendous stress of life-threatening illness, the anticipatory grief that it may engender, as well as the effects of both the disease and its treatment, may manifest themselves in cognitive impairments and psychiatric disturbance. Cognitive impairments such as forgetfulness, confusion, inability to concentrate, and poor concentration may be evident. Illness may reactivate earlier unresolved difficulties and may create such stress that the person's coping abilities are overwhelmed.

Psychiatric disturbances are also far more common in life among persons with life-threatening illness. One study (Hobbs, Perrin, and Irays 1985) for example, found that children with life-threatening illness are seven times more at risk for psychiatric disturbances than their well peers. Similarly, another study (Cyntryn, Moore, and Robinson 1973) found that 59 percent of a sample of cystic fibrosis patients had at least some degree of mental disturbance. Studies of persons who tested HIV positive (Buhrich 1986; Ostrow 1988) have identified a series of AIDS-related psychiatric syndromes such as dysphonia, phobias, anxiety disorders, and immobilization that follow diagnosis.

Suicidal Thoughts

The diagnosis of life-threatening illness, because it causes heightened anxiety for the survival and well-being of self and others, may well cause suicidal thoughts. If death is likely, an individual may reason, why not experience it now and avoid expected personal deterioration as well as the negative effects on family? Since suicidal wishes can be self-fulfilling, they should be resolved prior to surgery or other forms of treatment. The threat of suicide usually recedes in the early chronic phase after the crisis of diagnosis but may return with continued deterioration in the later chronic and terminal phases.

Hope

Hope usually exists throughout the experience of life-threatening illness. Many believe that hope can enhance coping skills and even influence survival. For example, Siegal (1986) emphasizes the importance of maintaining positive outlooks, believing that negative perceptions can become self-fulfilling. For Siegal the body and mind are inexorably intertwined; hope, strengthened through active imagining of the most positive outcomes, becomes a catalyst in achieving those desired results.

Throughout the course of the illness the focus of hope may change. In the prediagnostic phase hope usually centers on the symptoms either disappearing or having no serious significance. During the diagnostic or acute phase hope may center on the most optimistic outcomes, that the diagnosis will not be life threatening, for example, or that treatment will lead to cure or significant remission. Hope of cure or remission may continue throughout the chronic phase. In the latter periods of that phase hope may center on a slowed rate of deterioration or on a lessening of pain. In the terminal phase hope may center on surviving beyond significant milestones or events, or on the abatement of symptoms or pain.

Throughout periods of decline the time frame of hope will diminish. In the early phases of illness hope is likely to be expressed in years. In later periods that time frame may decline to days. "I hope to live to seventy years" may become "I hope to live to my birthday on Friday." In the early phases of illness hope is important because it encourages treatment and preserves self-identity and social relationships. In the terminal phase hope may focus on the afterlife or other modes of symbolic immortality, such as living on in the lives of descendents and a community, or in one's creations and accomplishments.

Emotional Responses

Guilt and Shame

Guilt and shame are common reactions to life-threatening illness. There may be "causation" guilt in which the individual feels guilty over personal behaviors or a life-style that may have contributed to the disease. For example, in one case an older man who had been diagnosed with throat cancer blamed his pipe smoking for the disease and felt very guilty that he continued to smoke despite previous warnings. Given the fact that many life-threatening diseases have behavioral components, this is not an unusual response.

There may also be "moral" guilt. Here the individual perceives the disease as punishment for some moral or character offense. For example, a person with AIDS may view the illness not so much as a result of having sex with an infected partner (which may itself create causation guilt), but as a punishment from God for what he believes to be sinful or immoral behavior.

While religious issues are often evident in moral guilt, especially in regard to diseases like AIDS where behaviors such as promiscuity and homosexuality face negative social sanctions, other issues may be involved. Many life-threatening diseases are often publicly perceived not only as lifestyle-related but also as character-related. A smoker with lung cancer may feel guilt both because he knows that his smoking contributed to the disease and because he has internalized social attitudes that smokers lack willpower. The guilt over the disease then moves beyond behavior to character. The cancer is seen both as a result of smoking and of the lack of enough will to stop. In other cases even the person's basic personality may be blamed for the disease. For example, explosive personalities may be seen as contributing to heart disease, while those who find it difficult to express emotion may be blamed for causing their own cancer. In fact, some nontraditional approaches to treatment emphasize that one must take resonsibility for causing the disease before one can hope to cure it. Caregivers need to be sensitive to the reality that one unfortunate by-product of theory and research on the psychological correlates of disease, and of certain treatment approaches that emphasize the individual's positive response to illness, is that disease victims may incorrectly internalize blame for their own illness. One study (Bennett and Bennett 1984, p. 561) emphasized that "excessive belief in the power of human influence over painful afflictions always carries a destructive potential."

In addition to moral and causation guilt, individuals may also exhibit a sense of "role" guilt. Here the focus of guilt is upon opportunities wasted and the limited time remaining. For example, an ill husband may feel guilty about past behavior to his wife. These feelings may even be exacerbated by the wife's support during the crisis. And he may feel guilty over the ways that his illness and perhaps death will affect his spouse's life. Role guilt can also be expressed as guilt over being a burden. Particularly in the chronic and terminal phases of illness, when one may require the intensive help of others, individuals may feel guilty about the demands they are making upon others and the ways that their illness is affecting the lives of others.

Anger

Anger is another common response to life-threatening illness. An individual is naturally angry that the illness is troubling his or her daily existence, complicating life and threatening possible death.

This anger may be directed at God. The individual feels outraged and cheated by the illness. There may be a sense of deep unfairness. "Why me?" is often an angry theme that emerges as persons cope with illness. For example, one young woman with cancer felt tremendous anger over the unfairness of the illness. She had two young children. She considered herself a moral person who had taken great efforts to lead a healthy life-style. Why me? and why now? were two big issues for her.

In other cases the anger may be directed at other individuals who can be blamed for the condition. In one case a worker blamed his employers for exposing him to hazardous chemicals that he believed were responsible for his cancer. In another case a woman who had contracted lung cancer was angry at her brother who had introduced her to smoking when they were both teenagers.

Sometimes anger may be directed at caregivers. One phenomenon that caregivers need to be aware of is "splitting." Here an individual's anger is turned toward one caregiver while others are excused from blame. Such scapegoating often exacerbates tensions among caregivers. Often the individual's false perception reinforces caregivers' self-concepts that they are just a bit more sensitive and skilled than others. It is important to recognize that client complaints even when focused upon one person may be a manifestation of an individual's anger over their illness.

Targets of anger can also include family and friends. An individual may become angry at his or her family, often because these targets are both closest and safest. Again, it is not unusual that one or two family members are scapegoated. One man with MS constantly focused his anger on his young teenage son. In counseling, it became clear that his anger tended to focus on the boy since he resented his son's growing vitality and emerging athletic powers just as his own mobility and physical state was so rapidly declining.

Friends too may become a focal point of anger and hostility. An individual may feel that friends are insensitive or unsupportive. While in some cases this may be true, in other situations friends are merely uncomfortable with or unable to respond effectively to the ill person's new, ambiguous status. The friend may also be receiving mixed messages about what the ill individual wants, needs, and expects.

Anger should be seriously evaluated and explored because sometimes it has a legitimate cause. Caregivers should beware of too readily dismissing anger. I once knew a chaplain who listened to a nurse's story about a patient who always complained about cold potatoes. The nurse suggested that this complaint really reflected the patient's anger at his illness. The chaplain asked the nurse if she ever put her finger on the potatoes!

While anger is a natural response, it can generate interpersonal tension, which both exacerbates stress and alienates crucial support. An individual's anger at the illness may cause him to strike out repeatedly at others in the immediate environment, often those very same people who are most needed to help in the struggle with disease. But anger can also be functional. Research (Weisman and Worden 1975) has indicated that persons who respond with anger and assertiveness tend to have longer survival rates.

Jealousy and Envy

Jealousy and envy are common human emotions, so common that two of the Ten Commandments address them. Jealousy and envy may be experienced by persons with life-threatening illness. An individual may be jealous of the good health of others. In some cases he or she may feel resentment of those who do not seem to appreciate their health, who misuse their time, or who lead lives perceived to be destructive. An individual may be jealous of other persons who seem to be responding better to treatment, coping more effectively with illness, or seemingly receiving more support. Family members may feel envious of other families untouched by illness, or by families that seem to be coping better. Because jealousy and envy are defined negatively, an individual or family may experience guilt over these emotions. Caregivers should recognize that these concerns are normal, and can help by encouraging individuals to review the ways that these emotions are influencing responses to illness and relationships.

Fear and Anxiety

The crisis of diagnosis produces fear and anxiety. Fears can include fears of the unknown, of loneliness, of extinction, of loss of family and friends, of the loss of body or mental functions, of loss of control, and of pain and suffering. In some cases fears will focus on what the disease and treatment may do to an individual's roles and identity. For example, an operation that mars the face may well cause anxiety about appearance and attractiveness that in turn will challenge identity. There may be fears the disease and its treatment will impair performance or make it impossible to maintain a career. Fears can focus on the operation or subsequent treatments; indeed, fear can be especially high prior to and immediately following surgery. Preoperative anxieties may focus on the fear of anesthesia, the loss of consciousness, or the effect of the operation (for example, causing additional damage, loss of organ and function, negative findings). Fears about postoperative care and life can focus on ability to function, employability, attractiveness, and finances. Postoperative anxieties may concern prospects for recovery; often anxious individuals will carefully scrutinize the remarks of physicians, nurses, and family for clues to their condition. There may be fears related to various therapies and their side effects. An individual may have fears that chemotherapy or radiation will cause sickness or sterility, leave him unable to function, or even create new cancer. Additional fears may focus on the fear of the dying process or on the ability of others to cope with the illness and possible death.

Fears and anxieties are likely to ebb and flow throughout the chronic phase. Often there is a persistent level of anxiety. During crisis points this anxiety can be intense. Even small events, such as the onset of a minor ailment such as a cold, can create great anxiety. Levels of fear and anxiety can continue even in cases of full recovery, often intensifying when illness or new symptoms threaten reoccurrence or perhaps when acquaintances suffer relapses or die of the disease. As the person approaches the terminal phase, anxieties may center on the process of dying (for example, the pain, dependence, indignity, loneliness); the loss of life (for example, separation, incompleteness, loss of mastery); the after-death (for example, fate of the body, judgment, the unknown); and the well-being of survivors.

Grief, Sadness, and Depression

Learning of life-threatening illness often generates feelings of grief, sadness, and depression. Sociologist Robert Fulton (1987) has described what he calls "anticipatory grief." Grief, he points out, is not only a response to losses one has experienced but also to those one *expects* to experience. In any life-threatening illness individuals and their families grieve both the losses they have already experienced, such as health, and the losses they anticipate, such as future declines in the health of an individual and perhaps eventual death. Similarly, Kubler-Ross (1969) described "depression" as being both reactive and preparatory. Reactive depressions are responses to losses already experienced while preparatory depression are reactions to anticipated losses.

These reactions can occur throughout the course of life-threatening illness, and are even common at the outset of such illness. For it is at the time of diagnosis that the person must first confront both her own vulnerability to disease and the possibility of further deterioration in health and eventual death. Sadness and grief reactions are also evident in the chronic phase. Here too people may have periodic bouts of depression, sadness, and grief, sometimes associated with clear crisis points. A bout with life-threatening illness heightens a sense of mortality and fragility even in the recovery phase. This "presentment" of death can also result in either ongoing or periodic depression. In the terminal phase, having already experienced significant losses (of health, of job, or mobility, and so on), and anticipating ultimate losses (of loved ones and life itself) depression, sadness, and grief are often experienced.

Depression may be manifested in a number of ways including constant sadness, fatigue, loss of energy, diminished interest in activity, insomnia or hypersomnia, and feelings of worthlessness. While depression is a natural response to life-threatening illness, it should be viewed seriously. Depression can sap energy for treatment, impair the quality of life, lead to suicidal acts, and perhaps even hasten death. Depressions that last over two weeks should be professionally evaluated and treated. Often antidepressants or therapy can be useful in mitigating depression.

Acceptance

Kubler-Ross identified acceptance as a common response to life-threatening illness, particularly in the terminal phase. Here the individual recognizes the inevitability of death and ceases to fight death. According to Kubler-Ross (1969, p. 113), "Acceptance should not be mistaken for a happy stage. It is almost void of feelings. It is as if the pain had gone, the struggle is over, and there comes a time for 'the new final rest before the long journey.' "

Acceptance can be a very complicated response. In some cases it may reflect the resignation that Kubler-Ross describes, while in others it may simply define an emotional collapse. Roberts (1988), basing her work on crisis theory, suggests that people unable to surmount the crisis of death experience a collapse of any remaining defenses. In still other cases death is ancticipated, that is, looked forward to, either as a release from pain and/or dependency or as an entry into a better and continued form of existence. And sometimes individuals actively acquiesce in death, even taking actions such as poor compliance to a medical regimen, refusing treatment, or even committing suicide. In summary, there are a variety of responses that may be identified as "acceptance" ranging from resignation to acquiescence.

It should also be noted that acceptance is not necessarily a desired state for all people. Such a position ignores the individual ways one faces death. Each individual has a different perspective on what constitutes a good death. Some may choose to struggle continuously against death, while others will almost rush to accept it. Sometimes acceptance can be premature. An acceptance response, particularly in the early phases of illness, may inhibit treatment and complicate any hopes for recovery.

Humor

Humor is one of our most basic coping mechanisms, one that can be very effective in times of crisis since it can release tension, ease stress, and strengthen social relationships. Sometimes it can even mitigate the shock of bad news, allowing individuals to regain their sense of control. Claire Kowalski, a dear colleague, composed this limerick at a time when she had heard some bad news:

> *A doctor I talked to this noon*
> *Forecast some dire symptoms quite soon.*
> *So I'll seek my own cure,*
> *And succeed to be sure,*
> *And that doctor can sing a new tune.*

Another limerick illustrates the way that humor allowed her to maintain hope and continue a positive outlook even in the midst of treatment.

> *This dear body on which I depend*
> *Is becoming my very best friend.*
> *So I'll treat it just right,*
> *Loving care day and night,*
> *And I know I am now on the mend.*

Another colleague facing ovarian surgery remembered that her last words to the doctor as she went under anesthesia were "keep the playpen." Norman Cousins (1979), in his book *The Anatomy of an Illness,* expressed his strong belief that his positive attitude and therapeutic use of laughter not only eased his adjustment to his illness, but was the key to his recovery.

Other Emotional Responses

Since illness and dying are processes of life, all the emotions experienced in life may be evidenced in life-threatening illness. There will still be moments of joy, happiness, and love. Sometimes such reactions can be experienced as part of the response to illness. Once a woman in the chronic phase of illness shared with me her joy and zest about being able to continue mundane household and work tasks that she had feared she might never be able to do again. Another client, faced with a continued decline, expressed his "unspeakable joy" at experiencing family moments and events.

Emotional responses, or any other pattern of responses, do not follow any order. And in any human situation, particularly a crisis, there may be considerable mood swings. One may feel depressed in the morning and feel much better by lunch. Often keeping a journal can be an effective way to monitor one's feelings and reactions throughout the course of an illness.

Behavioral Responses

Hypersensitivity

Persons with life-threatening illness may become hypersensitive. An individual often becomes extremely consicous of how others—family, friends, and medical staff—respond to him or her. He or she may exhibit great sensitivity to verbal and nonverbal behaviors of others. One woman, recovering from cancer surgery, for example, was convinced that her neighbors' use of paper plates at a casual barbecue indicated her fear of "catching" cancer from the woman who had cancer. An individual may scrutinize even casual remarks, especially those made by doctors and other caregivers, for clues about his condition, perhaps because he is suspicious that he has not been told the whole truth. A person may feel a need for continued reassurance that she is personally accepted, and of continued encouragement for treatment.

Persons suffering from AIDS are particularly prone to the problem of hypersensitivity. AIDS is a disease that many people fear, and it is associated with life-styles—homosexual, promiscuous, and drug-abusing—for which many people feel abhorence. Thus AIDS victims are twice-stigmatized: because they are diseased, and because of why they are diseased. Those who are infected with the HIV virus recognize that they are particularly stigmatized, and as a result they are quick to perceive slights from caregivers, family, or friends. This sensitivity can be seen even in the vocabulary of AIDS. Many people with AIDS strongly eschew the term "AIDS victim," preferring to be called PWAs ("Persons with AIDS") or PLWAs (Persons Living with AIDS). Similarly, attempts to distinguish some PWAs as "innocent victims" based on modes of transmission (for example, blood transfusions rather than sexual behavior or drug use) will be seen as highly insensitive by those who contracted the disease through sex or drug use.

Disengagement

Clinicians and researchers have long recognized that people often respond to life-threatening illness with disengagement, behavior in which they withdraw from others. Disengagement is often seen in the acute phase and also quite often in the latter period of the terminal phase.

The causes of disengagement can be quite diverse. In some cases it may be a manifestation of intense anxiety, pain, and egocentricity, all of which can cause people to withdraw from social interaction and focus on the self. In other cases it may be a symptom of underlying depression. In still other cases it may result from an intense involvement with inner issues and struggles. Finally, it may be a response to the isolation experienced when significant others—especially family and friends—withdraw from the ill individual.

Mastery and Control Behaviors

Someone who experiences life-threatening illness may have a strong feeling that his or her life is no longer in control. Not only are the ill facing an uncertain future, but they may be forced into a dependent role or they may anticipate future dependency. One way to respond to this loss of control is by trying to assert control even more strongly and attempting to master this experience.

These attempts at mastery and control can be expressed in a number of ways. One individual may try to learn as much as possible about his disease. Another individual may plunge into physical fitness activities, engaging in more-than-normal activity to reassure herself and others that she continues to function. Another person may seek cognitive control by intellectualizing the threat. Still another person may be very sensitive about maintaining personal control, for example, by carefully checking emotional expression. An individual may resist attempts by family, friends, and professionals to intrude on treatment decisions. Another person may assert control in the disclosure process. For example, an older man insisted that his wife keep the diagnosis from his four adult children, but over the next two days he individually shared that information with each child, swearing each one to secrecy.

Individuals may become assertive about their rights. For example, one researcher (Gustafson 1972) found that nursing home patients were insistent over issues such as new glasses or clothes since these struggles gave them a sense that they were still alive. In some cases people can become exceedingly manipulative, using their illness to obtain secondary gains. For example, in one case a young man attempted to use the fact that he had leukemia to maintain and control his relationship with his girlfriend. Whenever they had problems, he would insist it was because she could not deal with his disease, and he always added that a breakup would surely result in his relapse.

As with any response, these behaviors can be both appropriate and inappropriate. In some cases they can lead people to assume realistic responsibility for treatment. In other cases they can have negative implications, such as causing individuals to reject any dependent relationship, even one that might facilitate subsequent treatment.

Other problematic reactions include compulsive behaviors or counterphobic reactions in which the person asserts control through rejection of expert advice. Examples of compulsive behaviors include obsessions with health or adherence to particular rituals that an individual believes are associated with health. A diabetic adolescent who defiantly eats junk food and drinks beer would be an example of a counterphobic reaction.

Regression and Dependent Behaviors

Regressive and dependent behaviors are another response to the loss of control inherent in life-threatening illness. A person may respond to partial loss of control brought on by illness by surrendering additional control. Some psychologists suggest that persons typically respond to loss of control by making renewed efforts to exert control. Feeling that they are losing control, they try even harder to maintain it. However, if these efforts seem to fail, they may give up completely, allowing others to take even greater control of their lives than is necessary.

Overwhelmed by the diagnosis or by decline, some people regress and become dependent. This dependency can have other implications. Earlier conflicts over dependency, autonomy, and authority can reemerge. One older man, for example, who was struggling with diabetes, began to become very dependent upon his wife, asking her to monitor his diet, control his portions, and cook appropria te meals. However, at the same time he would sneak snacks and eat forbidden candies. In counseling, he recognized a similar pattern from his adolescence. As an overweight teenager he had expected his mother to help him adhere to his diet. But he also resented her efforts, and frequently sabotaged them. He realized he had transferred many of his unresolved feelings and behaviors from this earlier life experience to his current situation.

It is important for caregivers, both family members and medical staff, to try to emphasize, whenever possible, the autonomy of the ill person. While it often is easier for caregivers to do something for the ill person instead of leaving him or her to do it, each act may reinforce the person's own dependencies and lessened abilities. Often the line is difficult to draw, but individuals should be encouraged to do as much as possible.

Acting-Out and Resisting Behaviors

An individual may also respond to life-threatening illness by acting out and resisting behaviors. Displaced anger and hypersensitivity can lead to acting-out behaviors and increased interpersonal conflicts. People who are ill may be short-tempered and have frequent angry outbursts. Resisting behaviors, rooted perhaps in anger and denial, may be evident here as well, and may be manifested in such things as missed appointments, poor adherence to treatment, and counterphobic behaviors.

Transcendent Behaviors

Often feelings such as anger may be sublimated into more-acceptable behaviors, such as activism for a cause. For example, persons diagnosed with AIDS may join AIDS organizations designed to lobby for research monies or to focus attention on the problems of persons who are HIV infected.

Concerns about the meaning of life may encourage people to take actions that will utilize their remaining time to fulfill goals even if their activity exacerbates risk. For example, a woman with MS chose to have a child, even at the risk of further deterioration of her health, because being pregnant fulfilled a life goal and enhanced her sense of biological survival through an offspring. In another case a man diagnosed with Parkinson's disease decided to intensify his efforts to complete a doctorate. Thereafter, medical decisions and procedures took second place to his educational concerns.

In some cases individuals focus on assisting others. When one older man, for example, learned that he had a life-threatening disease, he became concerned about his wife's survival. She had a number of controlled chronic conditions that required a complicated medical regimen. He spent considerable energy on teaching his wife to be medically self-sufficient.

Still other people will show a renewed interest in religion and spiritual concerns. They may begin or intensify religious and spiritual activity such as attending church and praying. They may seek to complete or even repeat religious rituals. A formerly nonobservant Jewish man decided, for example, to have a bar mitzvah, even though he was fifty-seven. In another case a non-practicing Roman Catholic began to attend church once more, and even insisted upon a new baptism. People may begin to explore religious and spiritual books and theories. They may attempt various modes of spiritual healing from visiting shrines to laying on of hands to New Age techniques such as healing crystals. In some cases these can be attempts to make bargains with God or a defined "other power" for continued health and life. Often, such behaviors will be found early in the illness and will stop with continued deterioration. But in other cases these behaviors will continue or even intensify with deterioration. Such behaviors may reflect renewed interest and appreciation of spiritual and philosophical concerns, brought to the fore by people's struggles with their own mortality. It is important, however, that caregivers recognize that even though illness may awaken or intensify spiritual interests in some people, others may have a faith crisis. They may lose faith in a God that would put them through the suffering they are experiencing.

Coping Styles

The ways that we respond to life-threatening illness are often reflective of underlying coping styles. "Coping" refers to the process whereby one attempts to manage situations that place intense demands upon one's resources and anxieties. One's styles of coping include the affective, cognitive, behavioral, and spiritual ways that one characteristically uses in life. Psychologist Therese A. Rando (1984) makes a very important point that these coping styles are ways that one defends oneself against significant stresses and threats. Rando prefers the term "coping mechanism" to "defense mechanism," emphasizing the idea that the former term stresses the positive and adaptive aspects of coping rather than simply seeing it as reactive. Rando further notes that coping styles are neither unhealthy nor do they imply weakness. Rather, the ability to utilize effective coping mechanisms appropriately in the face of a major threat is a sign of emotional stability and health. Caregivers should support families' coping mechanisms, challenging them only when they are maladaptive. To Rando, maladaptive responses include anything that inhibits cooperation with treatment, increases the distress of illness, interferes with effective functioning in major roles, or creates psychiatric disturbance. I might also add to this list any behaviors that threaten the lives of others.

Rando describes three major patterns of coping:

1. *Retreat from the threat of death and conservation of energy.* Here individuals withdraw from interaction, become egocentric, exhibit a pronounced preoccupation with health, and regress. Such reactions are not necessarily problematic since they allow individuals to focus on their illness and receive help from others.
2. *Exclusion from the threat of death.* Here individuals cope by retreating from the threat of death. Among the coping mechanisms used are repression and suppression, rationalization, disassociation, and depersonalization.
3. *Mastery and control of the threat of death.* Here individuals attempt to control the illness by intellectualization, transcendence, sublimination, and varied forms of resisting responses.

Gullo and Plimpton (1985) divide children coping with life-threatening illness into six categories, each of which describes a strategic response to the threat of death;

1. *Death acceptors* confront their illness and possible death, accepting its reality and marshalling their resources (in a paraphrase of Saint Francis's prayer) to change and maximize functioning when they can and to accept with some serenity what they cannot change.
2. *Death deniers* cope with illness by denying its reality in the early phase of the illness and its gravity in the later phases. Even in the terminal phase they may insist that they will survive.
3. *Death submitters* collapse in the face of the threat of life-threatening illness and possible death. Feeling helpless and doomed, they put up no fight.

4. *Death facilitators* cope in ways that often seem counterproductive. They may fail to follow regimen and treatment, and they engage in risky behaviors that seem to invite death.
5. *Death transcenders* focus on other issues and all-but ignore life-threatening illness or possible death. Early in the illness they may focus on completing essential goals; later in the illness they concentrate on religious, spiritual, and philosophical concerns.
6. *Death defiers* fiercely fight the illness. Often these people exhibit much rage and anger.

Gullo and Plimpton's ideas about responses are similar to the ideas of Shneidman (1973). Shneidman was interested in intentionality, that is, the role that conscious or unconscious behaviors of people contribute to their own death. He notes that even deaths that are nonintentional still indicate varied responses toward death. And he further recognizes that many natural deaths may reflect a degree of ambivalence about life that Shneidman characterizes as subintentional. Shneidman's work on intentionality offers another way of viewing coping styles.

Nonintentional death are those where the person does not consciously or unconsciously seek death. These include:

1. A *death welcomer* plays no conscious role in death, but welcomes the end of life, perhaps as a release from suffering.
2. A *death acceptor* is passively resigned to his fate.
3. A *death postponer* tries to deny and hold off death as long as possible.
4. A *death disdainer* believes that death will not really come to him or her.
5. A *death fearer* is fearful and anxious about death. Often the death fearer will fight death, and deny and refuse to talk about it.

Subintentional Death is where an individual plays a part in his or her own death:

1. A *death hastener* unconsciously hastens death by refusing adherence to any medical regimen and by continuing a destructive life-style.

2. A *death facilitator* loses the "will to live," becoming a passive participant in death.
3. A *death capitulator* fears death so much that he or she almost seems to surrender to death.
4. A *death experimentor* takes chances with death by experimenting with medication or regimen.

Weisman (1986) describes fifteen common coping strategies employed in illness. These include:

1. Seeking information and guidance
2. Sharing concerns with others and seeking consolation and support
3. Laughing it off
4. Suppression
5. Diversion
6. Confronting the illness and acting appropriately toward the problem
7. Redefining the illness or crisis
8. Resigning oneself to the illness
9. Doing anything, even such things as substance abuse that exceed good judgment
10. Reviewing alternatives and consequences
11. Escaping
12. Conforming to what is expected or advised
13. Blaming someone or something
14. Venting
15. Denying

Weisman notes that many of these coping mechanisms might be employed throughout the course of the illness. For Weisman, adoptive coping mechanisms allow individuals to (1) confront the problem, revising plans when necessary; and (2) keep communication open and discriminately use the guidance and assurance of others. I might add another characteristic of effective coping that has been identified as a factor in long-term survival: (3) maintain a sense of optimism and hope.

In short, there are many different ways that we may cope with life-threatening illness because as humans we are unique and individual. Throughout the course of illness one may cope at different points in the illness in different ways. Many times, whether it is oneself or a family member who is ill, one may feel like one is on a roller coaster, sometimes up, sometimes down, other times flat. At each point in this roller coaster, one's own reactions and responses can be different. Throughout life one has developed a broad repertoire of coping styles. Different crises and different problems may call forth different responses.

One needs to understand that some of the ways we cope may help and hinder us at times. For example, a certain degree of dependency can facilitate adjustment, allowing one to accept help. However, too much dependency can sabotage one's rehabilitation at times when one may be expected to do more things for oneself. Similarly, coping styles that emphasize fighting and resisting disease may, many believe, increase survival time. But they can also create difficulties such as resisting needed help. There is also the risk of emotional collapse when these responses no longer seem to forestall deterioration or death.

It is important, then, to examine the ways that one copes with crisis. As I mentioned earlier, responses to prior crises in life can pinpoint strengths and forewarn us of possible problems.

Often it is helpful to talk with counselors, hospital social worekrs, or other caregivers. This does a number of things. First, one can clarify and explore one's feelings. Often one may repress many of the feelings one faces because they are so troubling. It may be hard to tolerate anger or jealousy or guilt. When one discusses these feelings, one can be reassured that they are natural and normal and find effective ways to resolve them. Second, one can reflect upon the ways that one is handling the illness and consider how to most effectively utilize one's own personal strengths and support. Counseling is often defined as help in crisis. There are few crises more severe than life-threatening illness.

Self-help groups of other individuals who share the illness can also be of great value. Shared stories of recovery or successful coping with disability can sustain hope. Members can support each other in crises, making one feel less isolated by realizing that others share similar feelings, reactions, problems, and concerns. Moreover, self-help groups can assist in solving problems by sharing solutions and strategies.

When one really understands one's responses, one can assess the way one's reactions and coping styles affect one's own sense of self, influence relationships with others, and complicate or facilitate the struggle with life-threatening illness. This may not only influence the quality of life, it may even change its quantity.

2

Understanding the Illness Experience

Death has been called "the Great Leveler." In many ways it is. We will all die: rich or poor, black or white, death is the common certainty. Nevertheless, life-threatening illness is affected by many factors. Our heredity, gender, social class, environment, culture, and life-style will influence how long we live, the illnesses we develop, the treatment we receive, and the ways we respond and react to the threat of illness.

Not only are the causes and course of life-threatening illness influenced by many factors, but the experience of illness is also very different for each person. Each illness is distinct, affected by the nature of the disease, the time in life when it strikes, and the circumstances that surround it. It is important to explore the unique experience of an illness, for such exploration enables each person, whatever his or her role—the person struggling with disease, a family member, a friend, or a caregiver—to understand and emphathize with the very individual problems and issues that the illness brings. This inhibits one for making unhelpful comparisons with how other individuals or family members dealt with illness. "Why can't she deal with it like Dad?" "How come I don't seem to have the attitude that served me so well before?" By recognizing the unique, personal experience of any encounter with life-threatening illness, we become better able to understand each person's response.

We will consider three critical factors in this chapter. First, every life-threatening disease or condition creates special concerns for the individuals it strikes and their families. Second, the time in the life cycle when a disease strikes also affects the experience of that disease. Third, an individual's life-style and personality influence his or her response to illness.

Disease-Related Factors: What Are the Particular Issues Raised by the Illness?

The Nature of the Disease

Where and how a disease manifests itself is often significant. Breast cancer, by its very nature, threatens sexuality and identity in ways that lung cancer does not. Breast cancer not only raises fears of possible death, but can undermine a woman's self-esteem, impair her sense of sexuality and attractiveness, and thereby affect her relationship with a spouse or a lover.

Any form of cancer can also leave strong fears about metastasis or reoccurrence, such that any subsequent symptom or pain will cause great anxiety. Any future cancer, even one that strikes years later and is unconnected to the first episode, may create a sense of hopelessness.

Other diseases raise their own particular issues. Many heart attack patients are left, even after recovery, with a heightened sense of vulnerability and anxiety that can permeate every activity and relationship. A friend of mine who suffered a heart attack now literally fears for his life whenever he faces serious stress. Similarly, those individuals who have experienced stroke may experience a reactive depression to any remaining physical or intellectual impairments.

Predictability of the Disease Course

Another factor that is important is the predictability of the disease. For some diseases both the prognosis and the probable course of the disease, including its timing are known, within certain limits. People with that disease are likely to have a specific life expectancy. In other cases prognosis, course, or timing may be uncertain. An example of the former kind of disease is pancreatic cancer. Here, there is a predictable likelihood that death will occur within a certain time range. An example of the latter kind of disease is multiple sclerosis (MS), which is characterized by great unpredictability. Some individuals with MS may decline rapidly while others will continue to function at high levels for decades. Uncertainty often makes illness more problematic to individuals and their families. This is often a key issue with AIDS, where there is a great unpredictability in symptoms and course. Persons with AIDS may have to cope with a wide range of symptoms. These symptoms can be both physical and neurological. The person may or may not experience viral infection of the brain, resulting in neurological impairment, personality change, or even dementia. From one day to another the AIDS victim may never know how the disease will progress.

Often the less predictable the disease, the more difficult it is to cope with it. When illnesses are reasonably predictable, everyone, including the ill individual, the family, and other caregivers, have clear expectations. Some kind of planning, however awful, can be done. When the disease has an unpredictable course, even this manner of coping is denied.

Symptoms

Different symptoms will also influence the experience of life-threatening illness. In some illnesses pain will be a constant, unwelcome companion, often affecting relationships and seriously impairing the quality of life. Diseases characterized by a persistent or disruptive set of symptoms can also create difficulties. For example, the constant coughing and wheezing and the foul-smelling stools characteristic of cystic fibrosis can lead to increasing isolation for its sufferers. Similarly, symptoms that are more visible can create a greater sense of stigmatization for those who are ill, for they feel more set off from the healthy than those whose disease does not include such obvious signs.

Psychological Effects

Manifestations of the disease can also differ in the psychological discomfort they can create for individuals. Threats to identity (for example, involving sexual organs or the face), colostomies, threats to mobility, loss of cerebral function, and specific critical incapacities (for example, loss of a leg for an active person) can be particularly distressing.

Diseases too have different meanings to different individuals. Because of past experiences or prior knowledge some individuals may have strong fears about a particular type of death. For some, cancer is the great fear, while others may fear a different disease. One gay man's first response to a doctor's prognosis that he could not survive his struggle with hepatitis B was "Thank God it's not AIDS."

Social Consequences

Different diseases also have different social consequences. Tuberculosis and cancer were once greatly feared. Today in our society AIDS generates such intense fear that persons with the disease are often isolated, stigmatized, and ostracized.

Disease Trajectory

Another important aspect of a disease is its trajectory or pattern. Glaser and Strauss (1968) describe the special issues each pattern has for individuals and their families. For example, a trajectory characterized by progressive deterioration and decline may cause different concerns than one characterized by remissions and relapses. The following trajectories create very different illness experiences:

> *The Gradual Slant:* In this trajectory one experiences a long, slow decline. Here the chronic phase may be quite long, often lasting years. Throughout this time the individual may continue to receive treatment, perhaps to retard gradual, progressive deterioration. The predictability often found in this pattern tends to create less anxiety and the evident gradualism tends to facilitate adjustment. However, the very length of the trajectory, particularly during the terminal phase, can create considerable stress for individuals and families. Often they may describe the illness as going on "too long."

The Downward Slope: In this pattern the decline is rapid, the chronic phase short or nonexistent, and medical treatment aggressive. Here the person must cope with rapid deterioration and the likelihood of death. Families must learn to cope with relatively sudden loss.

Peaks and Valleys: In this trajectory, exemplified by diseases such as AIDS or leukemia, there are alternating patterns of remission, relapse, and recovery. This pattern is characterized by considerable anxiety and constant stress, for often the timing of the relapses and remissions is unclear. Individuals and their families may not know how long a remission will last, how total recovery will be, or whether any given relapse will signal a final decline into death. Families may also experience the Lazarus syndrome where, because they expect the death of a person, they fail to adjust to that person's recovery and the continued repetition of the cycle.

Descending Plateaus: This pattern is characteristic of diseases such as MS. Here the person experiences declines, an indeterminate period of stabilization at that diminished level, then further decline and new stabilization. Like the pattern of Peaks and Valleys, this pattern is characterized by considerable uncertainty. One may not know how long a period of stabilization will last nor when a decline is likely to begin or how deep it will be. Unlike the Peaks and Valley pattern, however, declines tend to be irreversible, necessitating adjustment to a new level of disability.

Presentiment: This pattern characterizes persons who recover from sudden heart attacks or strokes. Here the recovery may be total, but the individuals and their families are very aware of their vulnerability to both subsequent reoccurrences and death.

Treatment Differences

Not only are the trajectory, nature, and symptoms of various diseases different, but their treatments differ as well. Treatment will have a significant effect upon the individual's experience of life-threatening illness. Three factors regarding treatment are important: the type of treatment, the nature of the treatment regimen, and the side effects and aftereffects.

Rando (1984) has described the psychological effects of different treatment modalities. For example, she noted that many people have considerable misconceptions and fears about surgery. Fears may be associated with the use of anesthesia and loss of consciousness, pain after the operation, or the visible scars resulting from surgery. Persons may be anxious about the extent of the surgery and the degree of dependence it may create both in the immediate postoperative period and later. They may also worry about the outcome of surgery, perhaps fearing that the surgery will not improve or may even harm their condition. In some cases surgery can even arouse other psychological issues such as feelings about guilt and punishment.

Long periods of bed rest following surgery or other special treatments may also have negative effects. Prolonged bed rest can adversely affect all the body's systems and create psychological difficulties, such as depression, decreases in problem-solving abilities, lessened motivation, and negative changes in body image.

Radiation may be feared because it is believed to be dangerous, perhaps even causing cancer, sterility, and other difficult side effects. Chemotherapy can raise similar fears.

The side effects and aftereffects of treatment will also influence the experience of illness. While in some cases side effects are minimal and barely disruptive, in other cases the side effects of treatment can be more devastating than the disease itself. Aftereffects too may vary. In some conditions the aftereffects of treatment are limited. Soon after the treatment stops patients can resume normal activities with little reminder of their ordeal. In other cases, though, the aftereffects can be lasting. Regimens too may range from simple self-monitoring of health to heavy, extensive, and burdensome regimens evident in diseases such as cystic fibrosis.

Individuals experience different reactions to treatments. Some people may be angry over the treatment or the resulting complications. Others may experience depression. In any case, every disease and every treatment creates different issues. The first step in understanding one's own or someone else's reaction is to consider the particular problems caused by this disease.

When Does Disease Strike? The Importance of the Life Cycle

While the characteristics of any given disease influence the experience of life-threatening illness, the experience is also affected by the time in life when that disease strikes. Illness is a different experience for adolescents than it is for older persons—not necessarily easier, but certainly different. At any point in life a disease brings up different issues as individuals respond both to the disease itself and to the different expectations and tasks of that phase of the life cycle.

Infancy and Early Childhood

There are a number of ways that life-threatening illness affects the young child. The intermittent periods of separation, the ever-changing environment, as well as painful and (to the very young) incomprehensible procedures may impair both the child's bonding and his or her development of trust. Periods of hospitalization can be particularly frightening since a young child may feel abandoned to strangers who cause pain. Many hospital programs now allow unlimited visitation by parents, including overnight stays, and encourage full parental participation in care and medication. This often mitigates some of the separation anxiety and isolation that children may experience during hospitalization. Parents may wish to ask about or even to suggest such programs if their infant or young child needs to be hospitalized.

Communication can be another major issue. Often parents of a young child are reluctant to inform the child about the disease or treatment. Their concern here is to protect the child and limit his or her distress. But often these attempts are counterproductive. Even young children will often be aware of the seriousness of their condition. This awareness can result from self-monitoring of their own condition, parental cues and responses, and comments from hospitalized peers. It is often less anxiety provoking to honestly answer a child's questions. Children will also find it comforting if they are prepared beforehand for any surgical or treatment procedures. Honest and open communication between parents and their children is effective in building and maintaining trust.

As the child continues to age and develop, the physical limitations caused by the disease and its treatments, and also by parental restrictiveness, may limit his or her ability to explore the world and develop autonomy. In addition, parental attempts to set limits and provide discipline, so critical at this stage, may be compromised by concern about the illness. Parents may be anxious and overly restrictive, sympathetically lenient, or seemingly inconsistent and arbitrary (based upon an assessment of the child's condition at that time). The result is that the child's developmental tasks of both exploring the environment and finding and recognizing limits are impaired.

While the child's ability to understand the reality of death or of life-threatening illness is a topic debated by many professionals, the differences between the parents' and the child's understanding of the situation as well as the anxiety generated in parents and children by the illness can complicate communication between parents and children. Parents may have considerable uncertainty about how, how much, and when to respond to their child's questions. The young child too may have considerable misunderstanding of the nature, cause, and treatment of the illness. Children often assume that illness is punishment for some offense. A five-year-old girl once told me that she thought she had cancer because she had left the gate open, allowing her mother's dog to escape to the street, where it was run over by a car. She was convinced that her illness was a punishment for her act and her later lies about it.

At any stage in their child's life, but particularly early in development, parents may also have intense anxiety about the long-term effects of both the disease and its treatment on subsequent development. They may worry that their child will have physical, social, psychological, or intellectual scars that may haunt the child's later life.

The School-Age Child

Life-threatening illness poses special issues for the school-age child. The child will need to learn to manage the illness within a school environment, which will cause him or her many problems. First, intermittent absences and the side effects of treatment can impair academic performance. Second, teachers sometimes assume that illness and treatment retard intellectual development, particularly if side effects include lethargy or confusion. Third, the treatment regimen may be difficult to manage within the classroom environment. Teachers may be resistant to interruptions posed by the need for medication or other aspects of treatment. School authorities may pressure parents to place their child in special education classes, an inappropriate classification for a child who can maintain academic performance, for such a reassignment can increase the child's sense of stigma and isolation, impair self-concept, and inhibit intellectual development.

Schools thrust the ill child into interaction with healthy peers, which can create other issuues. The stigma of the illness, limitations on activity, lack of self-confidence, and low self-esteem are but a few of the problems that can arise. In some cases other parents, afraid of the disease and overly protective of their own children, may discourage or prohibit their children from playing with the ill child. One study of children with cancer (Spinetta and Deasy-Spinetta 1981) found that they were more reluctant to participate in activities than their well peers. This in turn impaired subsequent growth and development. While teasing is a normal part of children's interactions with one another, such teasing can exacerbate the ill child's sense of being different, inhibit interaction, and lower self-esteem, especially since many ill children are already very sensitive and anxious about their disease.

Friends can share information that upsets the child. In fact, interaction with peers, either well peers or others with the same illness, in addition to increased access to both print and nonprint media that occurs at this age, make it highly unlikely that parents or other adults can successfully control the child's understanding of the nature or implications of his or her disease. Many of these problems can be mitigated by means of honest and open communication with the child and through the education of teachers and peers.

Illness complicates the struggles for mastery and independence typical of this age. Parents may be reluctant to allow their child necessary autonomy, thereby breeding overdependence. The child's own ability to master his or her environment may be affected either by the direct limitations of the disease or by an impaired self-concept. On the other hand, this natural desire for mastery can be well utilized, particularly within the chronic phase, by encouraging the child's increased responsibility and participation in treatment and treatment decisions.

The school-age child does face illness with two particular strengths. First, the child is often able to reach out for and to accept the help of supportive adults, something the adolescent may be more reluctant to do. Second, the child often firmly believes in his or her philosophy and faith, deriving comfort and strengths from those beliefs. The school-age child is more likely to ask "What is heaven like?" than to ask "Is there a heaven?" William Easson in his book *The Dying Child* (1970, p. 45) summarizes these strengths well:

> *The grade school child has the emotional ability to face the prospect of his death and to reach out to his parents and his family for comfort and understanding.*
>
> *Yea though I walk through the valley of the shadow of death . . . Thy rod and thy staff comfort me. This verse was written by a believer. These words could have been said by a grade school child.*

Adolescence

The key developmental issues of adolescence are often called the three I's: identity, independence, and intimacy. Life-threatening illness poses unique threats to each of these issues.

The adolescent's identity can be impaired in a number of ways. First, the physical deformities resulting from treatment of the disease may impair body image and self-concept. Second, these physical effects, associated limitations on activity, and periods of hospitalization can cause isolation from and rejection by peers, hampering self-esteem.

These same effects can also affect intimacy. The adolescent may be limited in his or her ability to establish ties with a peer group. As Easson (1985) notes, the limitations and disabilities caused by the illness may limit participation in and acceptance by more socially or athletically oriented peer groups. Or treatment and illness may retard academic progress, thereby limiting association and acceptance by more intellectually inclined groups. These same factors, he adds, limit the seriously ill adolescent's sexual outlets.

Illness is likely to complicate independence. If the illness begins in adolescence, the adolescent is forced into a more dependent role just at the time in the life cycle when he or she is trying to achieve a degree of independence. If the illness extends from childhood into adolescence, the adolescent may have already experienced a history of overprotectiveness that may result in a lack of early maturing experiences that increase passivity and impair the assumption of a more independent role. In both cases the uncertainty of the disease may limit and complicate planning for later adulthood.

The disease may face other difficulties as well. While adolescent conflict with parents is exaggerated, relationships with parents are often characterized by considerable ambivalence. This ambivalence, as well as the adolescent's quest for independence, may complicate the adolescent's ability to seek or to accept support from parents and other adults. Sometimes adherence issues can become a battleground between adolescents and their caregivers, reflecting the adolescent's need for independence and control. Allowing the adolescent to become a full partner in treatment by informing him or her about the need for adherence, tailoring the regimen to the adolescent's life-style, and soliciting the adolescent's participation in discussions and decisions can reduce that conflict.

In addition, adolescence is often a time of questioning beliefs. Thus beliefs about God and the afterlife that can be very comforting to the school-age child may provide less support to the adolescent.

The adolescent struggling with life-threatening illness also brings certain strengths to his or her struggle. Often their own resiliency and beliefs about personal indestructability can provide significant hope. Cognitive abilities and coping skills are more developed at this age.

Many of the negative affects of illness can be mitigated if those around the adolescent support the adolescent's individuality and independence. Recognizing that the normal needs of adolescence for autonomy and bonding with peers, as well as adolescent concerns about body image, often expressed in concerns about clothes and appearance, can help provide a sense of normalcy.

The Young Adult

Young adulthood is a time of looking outward, of beginning families and a career. Illness forces attention inward. As with the adolescent, then, illness during young adulthood can seriously affect the completion of tasks in the life cycle. It may impair independence and affect the development of relationships. It may introduce uncertainty to marriage and family plans. Disease may disturb the developing equilibrium between spouses, perhaps creating less-balanced relationships. It may have deep adverse effects on a career, impairing performance, limiting career mobility, perhaps even affecting employability and insurability. It may also influence financial planning and increase financial insecurity. Possible problems with insurance, the uncertain costs of illness, and unpredictable effects on future earnings may severely limit options at all stages of the life cycle. The thought of a limited life span may create deep anxiety and intense affect, and these issues may be intensified because everything the young adult has strived to achieve is now threatened.

The Middle-Aged Adult

Many of the same problems that plague young adults afflicted with life-threatening illness also trouble middle-aged adults. In some respects, life may have a more settled quality for those in middle adulthood. Jobs, careers, family, and friendship networks have probably stabilized. Yet life-threatening illness can unsettle all of these patterns. Relationships can undergo profound change. Career and financial stability may be jeopardized. Because financial and familial responsibilities may be at an apex in midlife, life-threatening illness can create great anxiety. And, as in early adulthood, it may also generate a strong sense of anger that one is being cheated so close to the prize.

It may also intensify normal developmental struggles. Midlife adults often develop an awareness of mortality, realizing that death is inevitable but still expecting it to occur decades in the future. This awareness, however, does intensify a desire to leave a mark, to pass on something to a younger generation. The psychologist Erik Erikson characterizes the challenge of midlife as "generativity versus stagnation." Life-threatening illness means that the awareness of mortality is not only future and abstract, but present and real. The man or woman whose illness threatens life may frenetically strive to accomplish all life goals even while struggling with disease. For example, in one case a teacher suffering from brain cancer insisted upon completing a master's degree and securing a job even though these goals added additional stress to an already stressful life. It was critically important for her to achieve these lifelong goals, delayed by the pressures of beginning a family, prior to her death.

The Elderly Adult

If the middle-aged adult is aware of mortality, the elderly are often described as aware of their own finitude. The older adult realizes the nearness of death, yet this awareness coexists with a continued sense of a personal future. While elderly persons recognize that they are approaching the end of their life span, they still may not envision their own personal death. Indeed, life-threatening illness may still come as a psychic shock.

The elderly have their own unique problems as they cope with life-threatening illness. First, this illness may come at a time when they are already coping with other chronic, although not life-threatening, illnesses. Thus their ability to surmount this illness may be threatened by their frailty. Second, their support systems may have been weakened by death or disability. They may lack able and appropriate caregivers. And they may worry about spouses or others dependent upon them. Illness may threaten their own caregiving responsibilities and heighten their fears for another's health, happiness, or survival should they become incapacitated or die. Third, many elderly people may ignore or discount serious symptoms since they believe that aches and pains are to be expected as part of the aging process.

Finally, there may be developmental difficulties as well. Developmental psychologists recognize that the elderly often undergo a life-review process, assessing their goals and accomplishments. Those who can say that their life had value, that they have accomplished much, can be said to have reached a state of ego integrity. Often this state makes it easier to face death. Perhaps the appeal of Frank Sinatra's song "My Way" is that it expresses that sense of having had a worthwhile life. In contrast, the person who feels that he or she has wasted life often spends his or her last days in despair.

This process of life review seems more related to a sense that death is near than to simple chronological age. For example, most dying persons will review their life as they become aware of death. Still, older persons may sometimes face unique issues that complicate this process. For example, the failures of children or the fact that they are the last of a name or line may be apparent only in later life, complicating life review.

Social and Psychological Factors

As I stated earlier, our response to and experience of illness is influenced by a variety of social and psychological factors. Among them are:

Characteristics such as Gender, Race, Ethnicity and Culture, Social Class, and Income

Social class and income level often affect the experience of illness. For example, persons of high social class have considerably more resources and therefore more options when coping with illness. I knew a young man of considerable means and impressive connections who developed cancer of the pancreas. He was able to parlay his contacts into referrals to expert physicians and participation in experimental treatment. Not only did special access probably increase his survival time, it also reinforced his ego at a critical time ("I can still make things happen"), and gave him and his surviving spouse a sense that everything that could be done was done.

Gender, race, and ethnicity also can influence the experience of illness. Longevity, causes of deaths, as well as responses to dying, death, and grief differ between sexes and ethnic groups. Even responses to caregivers and treatment may be influenced by these factors.

Intellectual Ability, Knowledge, Education, and Prior Experience

An individual's prior experience with disease as well as his or her knowledge, education, and intellectual ability can affect the experience of life-threatening illness. Previous experience with the disease, even if that experience is of limited relevance in the present context, can greatly influence the ways in which one perceives and responds to an illness. For example, a man who had suffered a heart attack at a relatively young age had considerable misconceptions and anxiety about heart disease, all rooted in his experience of his grandfather's disabling heart condition. In other cases, the experience with the disease may help us maintain more optimistic perceptions. A woman of my acquaintance who had breast cancer, for example, was deeply encouraged by two acquaintances' successful treatment.

Knowledge, education, and intellectual ability can have similar mixed effects. Individuals with higher levels of knowledge, education, and intellectual ability may be better able to relate to caregivers and take more participatory roles in treatment. But there may be negative factors as well. One nurse, for example, was aware of symptoms that she could associate with reoccurrence of cancer. Hence any such symptoms, even when these symptoms had clear alternate explanations, created intense anxiety for this nurse.

The Meaning of Illness, Life, and Death: Religious, Spiritual, and Philosophical Systems

Life-threatening illness is a crisis that has spiritual and philosophical dimensions since it raises questions about the reasons for illness, the role of suffering, and the meaning of life and death. Religious and philosophical beliefs and rituals can facilitate or complicate the spiritual struggle often associated with life-threatening illness. For some individuals, their religious or philosophical beliefs can be a source of great comfort. Belief in an afterlife may be a source of comfort and hope. Rituals too can be helpful. Prayer can be a highly therapeutic tool, allowing individuals opportunities to think about and share concerns.

But in other cases effects can be negative. Sometimes religious rituals can inhibit meaningful exchanges or convey unintended meanings to participants. One Italian Catholic mother I knew was enraged that her priest used the ritual "Anointing of the Sick" on her son, newly diagnosed with leukemia, since she associated it with the "Last Rites" and imminent death. And some beliefs may complicate the illness experience. A young gay man with AIDS was deeply troubled by his Fundamentalist background, for his childhood beliefs equated homosexuality with sin, punishment, and death.

Personality, Coping Skills, and Will to Live

In recent years considerable attention has been paid to the fact that personality, coping skills, and attitude are significant factors that affect not only the experience of illness but perhaps even survival time and survival rates. And while some question claims of longer survival, it seems evident that stress-resistant personalities, personalities that allow one to seek and accept help, better coping skills, and positive attitude can mitigate the great stress associated with life-threatening illness. It is also evident that medical staff respond differently to clients whom they perceive as having a "will-to-live," often intensifying their own involvement and efforts.

One's self-concept too is a critical factor in how one handles life-threatening illness. I have already discussed how a symptom of the illness or its treatment can pose a particular threat to a self-concept. Self-concept can also affect a person's ability to seek or accept help. One whose self-perception emphasizes independence and self-reliance may be unable to easily accept aid.

Informal Support: The Importance of Family, Friends, and Confidantes

Another critical set of variables influencing how we experience and respond to illness is the level of support we receive from family and friends. Supportive others can mitigate the stress of life-threatening illness in many ways, providing emotional support; assistance in daily living, particularly during the chronic phase; help in adhering to medical regimes; and other aid. Strong support from family and friends can help prevent a sense of hopelessness that may increase biological vulnerability and shorten survival time. Because the period of life-threatening illness can be long, and the care demands at times heavy, supportive networks that are both extensive (i.e., draw from a larger number of family and friends) and intensive (i.e., have members that are strongly tied to the patient) are best able to provide support. Not only are the quantity and quality of relationships important, but also the ways that family and friends relate. Relationships characterized by openness and honesty provide most support for individuals coping with life-threatening illness.

Formal Support

Formal support, or support from medical staff and other professionals, is another factor affecting how a person responds to and experiences life-threatening illness. Access to quality medical and nursing care can certainly affect survival time. But other forms of care such as social, psychological, and spiritual care can also influence both the quality of life and life length. For example, a recent study (Spiego and others, 1989) found that metastasized breast-cancer patients who attended weekly support groups lived longer than a control group that did not.

Concurrent Crises

Life-threatening illness is both extraordinarily stressful and self-absorbing. When this crisis is compounded by other crises, it may affect one's responses, strain coping resources, and inhibit support. For example, a woman with MS found her life greatly complicated when her husband had a car accident. Now he too needed care, just when her own mobility was limited. Many IV drug users with AIDS may also have chaotic and crisis-ridden life-styles that inhibit their ability to deal with their condition. Any ability to seek care and follow a complicated regimen is affected not only by low income, limited social support, and cognitive impairments associated with long-term drug use, but also by such crises as homelessness and arrests.

Summary

In short, anyone's experience of life-threatening illness and his or her response to it is highly unique and individual. It is affected not only by the distinct nature of the disease itself and by the time in the life cycle it strikes, but also by a range of psychological and social variables. A key concern is to examine these factors to understand how they complicate or mitigate the experience of illness.

3

Understanding the Road Before

One's confrontation with life-threatening illness or death can develop in a number of different ways. Often it may result after one seeks medical advice and treatment in response to the appearance of a troubling sign such as a lump in a breast or blood in the urine. In other cases it may result from the confirmation of a positive test result, such as an HIV antibodies test or a tuberculin test. Such tests may have been sought even though one was asymptomatic because one engaged in at-risk behaviors, suspected exposure, or simply sought reassurance. In still other cases the encounter with illness may be sudden, as with the experience of a heart attack or a stroke. Finally, the encounter may come about as an unexpected result of a routine physical examination or test that reveals an unsuspected serious illness.

We often consider the beginning, or acute, phase of illness to start with the diagnosis of illness. In reality, the encounter with life-threatening illness often predates the diagnosis. No matter what the circumstance of the encounter, there may well be a period prior to one's certain knowledge of illness during which one struggles with suspicion of illness or knowledge, at some level, of risk. Whatever the circumstances that lead one to the fateful moment of diagnosis, it is useful to understand our behavior in the process that preceded it. Making decisions to seek medical help—"health-seeking" as it is sometimes called—is a complex process that can often tell much about how we will respond to the crisis of illness.

Tom's case illustrates this point. Tom, a man in his fifties, had been having problems with urination for a few months. For a long time he simply ignored these problems, even neglecting to mention it to his physician during a routine visit. After a while he began to tell some friends about his problem, and they had the wisdom to advise him to seek medical help. When he did, tests indicated a growth on his prostate gland. His delayed health-seeking almost cost him his life!

Understanding the process of how we seek medical health should provide opportunities for growth rather than guilt or blame. Reviewing one's behavior prior to diagnosis can reveal one's fears and anxieties, coping mechanisms, and sources of support. Tom, for example, recognized after the fact that he had suspected cancer all along. He knew, based on his own previous experiences with his father's death from cancer, how much that possible diagnosis frightened him. His new experience with disease taught him that he had a strong tendency to deny and avoid things that made him anxious. Realizing this characteristic helped him and his physician throughout the course of Tom's successful treatment. As a result of his illness, Tom also could identify the friends and family members with whom he was comfortable discussing his illness. He found, much to his surprise, that he had tried to shield and protect his wife, but that he was comfortable discussing his anxieties with a few close friends.

There is much value in understanding the ways one behaves prior to diagnosis. Each person may follow a different path to that diagnosis. In each case, though, it is worthwhile to review the context and circumstances that led to this moment of crisis.

One of the most common contexts, and certainly one of the most researched, is when a person learns of a life-threatening illness while seeking medical attention for a troubling symptom. Medical sociologists have long recognized that seeking such treatment is a complex process influenced by many factors. This process provides a model for the factors that characterize health-seeking even in other situations.

Symptoms of illness, especially at their onset, are rarely so dramatic or unambiguous as to mandate immediate attention. There is often a period of delay during which these symptoms and their implications are interpreted and evaluated by the person so afflicted. In some cases this period of delay can be so long as to imperil any opportunity for successful treatment.

The evaluation of symptoms is likely to be influenced by four sets of factors: symptom-related factors, physical and psychological factors, situational factors, and social factors. (This section draws from the work of Bloom [1965], Coe [1970], Davis [1972], Dingwall [1976], Harowski [1987], Spector [1985], and especially Mechanic [1968, 1980].)

Symptom-Related Factors

Often the very nature of the symptom will be a major factor affecting the person's decision to seek assistance. Symptom-related variables include the following:

How Apparent, Recognizable, and Serious Are Symptoms?

Symptoms that are more apparent, such as sharp pains, fever, rashes, are more likely to command attention than those that are less apparent, such as a general malaise. Similarly, symptoms that are more recognizable and considered serious by most people, such as blood in the urine or stool or a lump in the breast, are apt to receive more consideration than vague feelings of fatigue or soreness.

The more a symptom is considered to be a sign of future danger, the more likely action will be taken. While a lump in the breast can be many things, many of which are harmless, most women recognize such a lump as a possible sign of cancer. On the other hand, a backache can also foretell serious illness, but is often perceived as far less worrisome.

How Disruptive Are the Symptoms?

The more a symptom disrupts family life, work, or other social activities, the earlier action is likely to be taken. A persistently painful toothache demands a quick trip to a dentist. A less-disruptive symptom that does not impinge on one's personal or social life may not be as pressing.

How Frequent and Persistent Are the Symptoms?

Symptoms that are perceived as both less persistent and routine may not receive the same concern as those that are persistent and/or recurring. In the former cases, it is easy to wait out the symptoms, hoping they will not reoccur.

Possible Alternative Interpretations

When an alternate explanation exists for a symptom it is often less worrisome than when an appropriate explanation is not available. A lump that follows trauma is often perceived as less frightening than one that simply appears "on its own." Similarly, fatigue or aches after vigorous activity are perceived as less troubling that those that lack explanation. When one can rationally account for symptoms, one typically feels less concern.

Part of the evaluation of explanations also includes a strong sense of personal biography. "Am I a person who is vulnerable to this disease?" is often part of the interpretive process. For example, a man with a family history of coronary disease may well perceive chest pain differently from one who has no such history. An active homosexual may respond with panic to a night sweat, a possible indicator of AIDS, while someone not at risk might consider the symptom of little consequence. A person who has recovered from cancer may be far more sensitive to signs or symptoms that might suggest possible relapse.

Physical and Psychological Factors

In addition to the nature of symptoms, other factors such as physical and psychological states affect both the evaluation of symptoms and the decision whether to seek medical help. Among these are:

Tolerance Thresholds

Individuals vary in their assessment and toleration of pain and discomfort. Sometimes our cultural background affects our experience of pain. One study (Mechanic 1980) found that persons of Irish and English extraction tended to have higher levels of pain toleration than a sample of Jews and Italians. Men are less likely to complain of pain than women. Individuals also may differ in their pain thresholds. The point is that for a variety of physiological, cultural, and gender-related reasons, pain or symptoms that may send one person for medical attention may be tolerated by others.

Basic Beliefs and Knowledge

Another variable that effects health-seeking is a person's basic belief systems. Basic to seeking medical attention are the beliefs that one is susceptible to disease, that disease states are harmful, that intervention can help, and that assistance is therefore worth seeking. But not everyone accepts the modern scientific theories that underlie disease diagnosis and treatment.

Social and cultural beliefs about the type of treatment that is suitable can also affect the health-seeking process. Every culture has beliefs about illness causation, treatment, and referral. For example, in a cultural system dominated by folk beliefs, an ill person will probably turn to folk practitioners before seeing a physician. In other cultures outside treatment may always be sought within the medical system.

Knowledge too is a variable. Individuals may differ in the degree to which they recognize the significance of symptoms. This may affect the process of seeking treatment. A person who recognizes that numbness is a sign of multiple sclerosis will be more likely to seek help for that symptom than one who does not have that knowledge.

Anxiety Level

The level of anxiety produced by the symptom is also a factor in seeking assistance. Any symptom can generate considerable anxiety. The anxiety may result from a number of concerns including the nature, difficulty, and process of diagnosis and/or treatment; the humiliation, embarrassment, or stigma associated with the symptoms or suspected disease; and fears related to coping with the treatment such as anxieties about surgery, concerns about childcare or work, or worry about finances. Maria, for example, an older Italian woman, delayed seeking attention for a lump in her breast because of embarrassment, while Mark, a thirty-year-old businessman, neglected chest pains because he feared hospitalization would affect his work schedule.

Not only are levels and sources of anxiety likely to differ among individuals, but ways of coping with anxiety may vary as well. In some cases anxiety can distort the perceptual process of evaluation. For example, the level of anxiety may be so great that an individual like Tom will deny the symptoms. Behavioral responses may differ as well. The anxiety experienced by some individuals inhibits them from seeking medical attention, while the anxiety felt by other individuals actually compels them to seek help.

Personality Characteristics

Other personality characteristics, such as one's willingness to disclose information about one's self, or how extroverted or trusting one is, are among the factors affecting the health-seeking process. Seeking medical assistance is often a later step in a process that involves both self-appraisal and discussions with family and friends. I will describe this process in greater detail later; here it is important to note that varied personality characteristics, such as low self-esteem, introversion, introspection, and a lack of trust and/or self-disclosure, may inhibit or distort this process. For example, people who are very private about their affairs may find it hard to consult others, whether professionals or their intimates, about troubling symptoms. Similarly, persons who are highly introspective are more likely to be aware of bodily sensations and physical symptoms than those who focus their attention outward.

Childhood Experiences

Developmental experiences also seem to play a role in the evaluation of symptoms. Early experiences with illness may make us more sensitive to symptoms and more acutely aware of bodily sensations. An adult who experienced rheumatic fever as a child may recognize a vulnerability to heart disease and therefore be more attentive to suspected heart-related symptoms. These experiences may be indirect as well. Persons who have witnessed the illness of a significant other may be more aware, attentive, and anxious regarding similar symptoms in themselves.

Parenting styles too may affect health-seeking behaviors. A study of young adults (Mechanic 1980) found that those who had experienced abusive parenting tended to report and to monitor physical symptoms more closely, suggesting that this attitude may have resulted from additional stress or more introspection that this early abuse seems to engender. As I stated earlier, this introspection often leads to greater attention to one's physical state.

Situational Factors

Social Context

Individuals' evaluations of their physical states are also influenced by the larger social context. For example, health campaigns or portrayals of illness in the mass media can make the public more aware of certain diseases and thus more attentive regarding its symptoms. Epidemics can sensitize people both to the significance of symptoms and to the likelihood of possible infection. For illustration, one study (Davis 1972) showed that during the polio epidemic parents were much more likely to call a doctor even though they believed their child only had a cold; because they were aware of polio cases in their area, they were more sensitive to their child's potential vulnerability to polio. Similarly, as the AIDS crisis unfolded homosexual men were far more attentive to rashes and other symptoms than they had been before. Some, in fact, search their bodies daily for evidence of rash.

Competing Needs

I once saw a humorous wall plaque that stated "Once the busy season ends, I'm going to have a nervous breakdown—I'm entitled." In a sense, that joking statement points out the impact of the environment on health-seeking. At times when many needs compete for one's attention, only the most sustained and serious symptoms will get attention. There are a number of reasons for this. First, one's attention is generally focused outward; therefore physical sensations are likely to get less attention. One tends to focus on inner states only when the distractions from the external environment are minimal, or conversely when internal physical symptoms are so overwhelming that one can no longer function. Second, a number of symptoms such as fatigue, headaches, or soreness can be attributed to the press of external circumstances, and therefore discounted. Third, seeking medical evaluation and treatment often has a lower priority than immediate pressing problems.

Availability of Help

Ease of seeking assistance can also be a factor. This has two elements. People are likely to seek out family and friends first. They may want to discuss and to compare symptoms with others whom they know and trust. This process will also be facilitated when those available to consult are perceived by people as being similar to themselves. Thus, access to others to whom one is close can sometimes facilitate the health-seeking process.

Second, the accessibility of formal medical assistance will also be a factor. Easy access to appropriate medical help, unrestricted by financial, linguistic, class, or geographic barriers, will make it more likely that a person will seek such help.

Social Factors

The previous discussion should make clear the importance of other social, intervening variables such as culture, social class, gender, age, and education. All have direct as well as indirect impacts on health-seeking.

Culture

Our behavior is always influenced by our culture. Culture frames one's entire belief system about the nature and cause of illness, the efficacy of treatment, even the process of seeking outside assistance. For example, in some cultures traditional healers may be consulted instead of or prior to turning to the medical establishment. In addition, linguistic or cultural barriers may inhibit both the process of health-seeking and subsequent treatment.

Social Class

Social class too can have a significant impact on health-seeking. For example, some observers believe that low-income persons are often fatalistic and present-oriented. Low-income persons may feel that they have little control over the future; in any case, the problems of the present are so overwhelming that the individual has no energy left to address the future. In one case a lower-class woman with a family history of cancer who had a lump in her breast was urged to see a physician. She resisted, claiming that "It wouldn't make any difference." Even when convinced that medical care could help her, she repeatedly missed appointments both to take the cancer test and then to discuss the results, each time claiming a sudden family crisis or lack of funds. When the test results proved to be positive, she responded, "I was born under an unlucky star," and the pattern of missed appointments continued thereafter throughout her treatment.

Similarly, low-income people may have ambivalent attitudes toward authority figures who are likely to differ from them in terms of educational levels and language. This problem can affect doctor-patient interaction, limiting the person's disclosure of illness, and complicating a health professional's understanding of a client's description of symptoms. Social class will also have a direct impact on the accessibility of help and an indirect effect of education.

Educational Level

A person's level of education has a clear relationship to his or her understanding of symptoms and sources of help. As I stated earlier, disparities between the educational level of the patient and health professionals may inhibit the communicative process.

Gender Roles

Gender roles also seem to be a significant variable in health-seeking. First, there are differences between the sexes both in longevity and causes of death. These differences may affect the way an individual perceives risk and responds to symptoms. Second, as part of the traditional male role, males are taught to minimize and to ignore minor physical symptoms. There is also evidence that male doctors may not perceive certain female symptoms such as morning sickness or menstrual cramps as serious.

Age

Age also affects the evaluation of medical symptoms. First, standards of health differ by age. An acceptable blood pressure for someone fifty years old is far different than that for someone five years old. Second, the perceptions of both health professionals and patients themselves may be influenced by the age of the patient. For example, an elderly person may be more likely than a younger person to ignore symptoms by attributing them to age; of course, this attitude delays diagnosis. Similarly, health professionals may also discount the symptoms of an elderly person.

Other Social Roles and Behaviors

Other roles can influence perception and evaluation of symptoms. For example, even prior to the AIDS epidemic promiscuous homosexuals were aware of their vulnerability to a number of sexually transmitted diseases. Certain occupational groups, such as coal miners, are often aware of potential occupational diseases and may be especially attentive to symptoms. As I stated earlier, such attentiveness may be particularly acute when media attention or personal and group experiences cause one to focus on a particular illness. Religious beliefs too have been identified as influencing health-seeking. For example, religious beliefs might influence attitudes about the illness and treatment (God's will) that inhibit health-seeking or they might suggest alternate treatment, such as prayer, pilgrimages, religious healers, and the like.

The Process of Health-Seeking

In summary, the process of seeking attention for a troubling symptom is complex, multifaceted, and influenced by many things. I can use gestalt psychology to illustrate this process. A basic gestalt premise is that one often ignores the ground and focuses on the "figure." In health-seeking this means that one tends to ignore internal states until conditions force one to respond to them either because the internal stimulus, such as pain, becomes so intense that it mandates a response or because circumstances in the external environment continually redirect one's attention to that internal state. In short, then, one's attention is normally directed outward, but some conditions will cause one to pay attention to bodily sensations and symptoms. Once that attention is redirected, it can create a great deal of anxiety and concern.

At that point, the person experiencing these symptoms may have to formulate both an evaluation of the symptoms and a response. People may interpret a symptom as normal and ignore it, or they may determine that information is incomplete so they decide to wait and see. Or they may judge the symptom as abnormal. Even in that case the responses can be different; possible responses include ignoring the symptom, treating it one's self, or seeking some form of assistance. This process of evaluating symptoms and responses is ongoing. Evaluating symptoms is a constant process of hypothesis testing. One's tentative diagnosis is constantly evaluated in the light of new evidence. For example, a lump or a bruise may first be defined as normal. However, if it grows, or does not heal within a certain time frame, or if it changes in some way (such as becoming more painful), a new tenative conclusion may be drawn. Fred Davis (1972), in his account of the polio epidemic, offers further illustration. Some parents initially perceived the symptoms of polio as a cold. When their child failed to get well, the parents wanted to believe that the child was malingering. But when the child continued to get sicker, their earlier hypotheses no longer held and parents were forced to recognize the possibility of polio.

This process is also likely to involve consultation with others around us. A person experiencing a symptom may ask family members and friends for their evaluation of the symptoms, and also ask for their advice about treatment. In situations where the symptoms are visible, or when they impinge upon behavior, family, friends, and others may offer unsolicited advice. Thus there may be cycles of assessment, reassessment, and treatment that only after time may culminate in a decision to seek medical treatment.

Health-Seeking in Other Contexts

Not everyone finds out that they have a life-threatening illness when they seek evaluation of a troubling symptom. Some may learn of the illness even though they have no symptoms. This may occur in the course of a normal physical examination. Still, my previous discussion of health-seeking is relevant here too, for a process may precede such testing.

Often someone has elected to take such a test, even though he or she is asymptomatic, because he or she fears exposure to the disease. In that context, clinicians may believe that a positive result would not be a complete surprise to the client.

Yet limited research on the HIV antibodies test casts doubt upon this assumption. A person's motivation for taking the test as well as his or her perception of risk can vary considerably. In some cases there is a high perception of risk, while in other cases there is no real expectation of a positive result. People may take the test because they are beginning a relationship, recovering from addiction, ending an infidelity, having a routine insurance physical, or making a political statement (for example, supporting an ex-addict or gay organization's call for testing). Such people may have every expectation that the result will be negative.

Even in these situations it is helpful to explore such issues as the individual's assumptions, motivations, anxieties, and expectations about the test; their knowledge, beliefs, and experiences about the disease and treatment; and their process of deciding to seek both the test and results. While this counseling has become relatively common with HIV testing, it is not common with other tests for life-threatening disease.

Evidence of life-threatening illness can also be found by means of routine tests and procedures. For example, a blood test may find chronic lymphocytic leukemia or suspicion of another serious illness even though the person is asymptomatic. Similarly a blood donation may test positive for the HIV virus. In these cases, the shock of life-threatening illness is compounded by the individual's lack of perception of risk.

Nonetheless, it is valuable to explore the motivations, behaviors, and anxieties preceding even these tests and examinations. Was this simply a routine physical, continued monitoring of a prior recovery, or was there a suspicion of illness? How often and under what circumstances does the person normally get examined? What was the process preceding this physical? For example, delaying and resisting or missing appointments preceding the physical may indicate anxiety and/or denial and may be a cause of subsequent guilt. What are one's feelings prior to a physical in general, and toward this physical in particular? Some may approach a physical with a sense of anxiety while others have no such feeling.

There are causes in which one encounters life-threatening illness or conditions that do not seem to involve any conscious decision on one's part to seek help. In these cases one is suddenly and dramatically thrust into the situation. With a heart attack or a stroke, for example, one is quickly and unexpectedly made aware of one's own fragility and vulnerability.

But even in these cases it may be worthwhile to consider prediagnostic behaviors and attitudes. Was there any suspicion or evidence of problems? Was there any expectation of risk? Could and did one at some time perceive a risk (for example, high blood pressure, obesity, or the like)? What was prediagnostic behavior? Had friends and family expressed concerns?

Understanding the road ahead is critical. Whether one realizes it or not, one has completed three tasks. First, one recognized, at some level, a possible danger or risk. Second, one began to cope with all the anxiety and uncertainty inherent in that danger. Third, one developed a plan of action to deal with that concern. By reviewing and exploring that process, a person—whether the ill individual or a family member—not only knows where he or she has been but how he or she got there. We can understand and use the strengths we have uncovered and compensate for the weaknesses we have discovered. We can use that knowledge to grow and meet the challenge of other tasks throughout all the remaining phases of life-threatening illness.

The Crisis of Diagnosis

The Diagnostic Divide: The Acute Phase

Whatever symptoms or suspicions may exist in the prediagnostic period, whatever fears are entertained, the diagnosis of life-threatening illness always comes as a shock. Anthony Ferrara, a psychologist who later died of AIDS, captured the moment well. Though he suspected the spots on his skin were Kaposi's Sarcoma, an almost sure sign of AIDS, he was still stunned and overwhelmed at the actual diagnosis (1984, p. 1285): "All of my mental preparation was insufficient to thwart the tidal wave of emotion that swept over me as I received what at the time I regarded as a death sentence."

Until the actual diagnosis, no matter what the expectation, suspicion, or fear, there is always a chance that any self-diagnosis might be a mistake. The lump may yet turn out to be a benign cyst, the rash to be only a minor problem. This thinking changes at the time a diagnosis is rendered. Here one's worst fears are realized and the person is forced to recognize that he or she is now either in a struggle for life or an inexorable slide toward death.

The time of the diagnosis is often described as a turning point, a time of crisis when one's whole orientation toward life changes. According to Weisman (1980), this confrontation with possible death overwhelms people, creating the shock and numbness that he terms "impact vulnerability." For Weisman, diagnosis is a time of "existential plight" during which one must cope with the crisis of possible death. Many psychologists emphasize that a diagnosis of life-threatening illness is second in causing stress only to knowledge of dying itself.

It should be recognized that the time of diagnosis is often not a simple moment, though it may culminate in that moment when the diagnosis is spoken. Rather, it is a process unfolding over time in which a person experiences various tests or procedures during which different hypotheses of illness are advanced and sometimes discarded.

The process of rendering a diagnosis is often very difficult. During this time people may have to cope not only with a multiplicity of medical tests and procedures but also with a great deal of uncertainty. During this period an individual may be asked to take numerous diagnostic tests. Some of the common tests include:

X-rays—Used to look into the chest or to check for broken bones

CT Scan (Computed Tomography)—A type of X-ray that uses computers to produce a cross-sectional picture of the body

MRI (Magnetic Resonance Imagery)—Similar to a CT scan; here a computer image of the body is constructed by using a magnetic field

Angiograms, Radioactive Isotopes, and Ultrasound—Approaches that allow physicians to view the inside of the body, enabling doctors to track blood vessels or to view organs and tissues

Electrocardiogram (EKG, ECG, Cardiogram)—Allows physicians to monitor the electrical impulses of the heart to diagnose heart disease

Spinal Tap (Lumbar Puncture)—Allows physicians to withdraw and study cerebrospinal fluid, which can reveal the presence of a variety of different conditions

Blood or Urine Tests—Useful in a variety of circumstances: to test for antibodies, to discover infections, or to monitor body chemistry

Biopsy—Tissue is removed from the body and examined. A biopsy is the only way to confirm a diagnosis of cancer; only by examining the tissue itself can physicians determine whether the growth is benign or malignant.

In addition, there are many other diagnostic tests specific to a certain location of the body, such as a brochoscope that examines the bronchi, a section of the lungs, or for identifying a targeted condition. Your physician should explain to you the purpose of the tests, the procedures involved, when results will be available, and how they will be communicated to you.

It is important to remember that many of these tests are part of *a process of diagnosis;* any one test may not be definitive in and of itself. For example, if physicians suspect a tumor they may wish to perform a variety of tests such as a blood test, a CT scan, an MRI, and other tests to locate and assess the nature of the tumor. But only a biopsy will tell them if the tumor is cancerous. Subsequent tests, called staging tests, may be required to see how advanced the cancerous condition is. Similarly, if a person tests positive for HIV antibodies with an initial ELISA test, physicians will generally retest with a more accurate Western Blot test. Some people who test positive with the former test may not show evidence of HIV antibodies on the latter test. And even if both results are positive, further blood tests may be necessary to assess the stage of HIV infection.

Diagnosis is a process during which physicians test their hypotheses, when varied explorations are evaluated against emerging information. Throughout this period the individual being tested will experience wide mood swings as a continuing flow of information changes both the possible diagnosis and the prognosis. For example, in my father's case, the initial symptom was blood in the urine. While this physical fact stimulated great concern, we recognized that numerous conditions, some of which were minor, could account for the blood. Subsequent examinations led to the suspicion of a mass on both the kidney and the pancreas. More tests pinpointed the growth on the gall bladder and kidney. Surgery successfully removed both tumors; one was encapsulated; but the other was unrelated and benign. During the course of the week when the testing and surgery took place, my father's prognosis changed from uncertain to poor to hopeful to excellent. The moods and reactions of my father, our family, and even the physician changed in tandem with the emerging diagnosis.

One always has to remember that diagnosis is as much an art as a science. Most life-threatening diseases have some degree of uncertainty. Many diagnostic tests really do no more than point to the *probability* of a certain result. At each successive level of testing, however, the diagnosis may become more certain. But even then the course of the disease—how the disease will unfold and develop—still may be uncertain.

Not only is the diagnosis characterized by at least some degree of uncertainty, the prognosis often has considerable uncertainty as well. Assuming that the diagnosis is as accurate as the process allows, numerous other variables can affect prognosis. Diseases themselves may differ in the degree that prognosis is clear. An individual's health, attitude, and adherence to the medical regimen; the nature of care; the effectiveness of varied therapies; the stage at which the disease was discovered; the impact of subsequent medical progress—all these factors can influence prognosis. It is important to remember that any prediction is at best a statistically grounded estimate, perhaps only loosely based upon relevant variables and the current state of ever-changing medical knowledge and treatment. For many people these predictions can be useful. They may allow all those concerned to envision a sense of time that will facilitate planning and assist individuals and families in evaluating different options. But no prediction should ever be considered certain. Almost every family can offer anecdotes about family members who not only outlived predictions, but sometimes even the physicians who made them.

The diagnosis of life-threatening illness creates an intense crisis filled with anxiety, strong emotional reactions, and many personal and interpersonal issues. Tensions and anxieties mount. Individuals must either learn effective ways of coping or experience personal disorganization and intense anxiety. The very knowledge of life-threatening illness results in intense crisis for newly diagnosed persons and their families. The fact of illness is beyond one's control. Yet the diagnosis of illness affects the whole family: all family member goals, all family member roles, and all family member relationships. Despite this crisis of uncertain nature, everyone in the family has to make a series of initial decisions that well may radically affect the quality, nature, and even duration of a loved one's life. Life-threatening illness has ramifications that affects every aspect of life: relationships with families and friends, financial decisions, work, and school. In fact, virtually

all plans will need to be reevaluated in the new context of diagnosed illness.

Throughout this period a number of issues are raised for the
person who is coping with the diagnosis. These may be viewed as
tasks that the person must consider. These tasks include:

1. Understanding the disease
2. Examining and maximizing health and life-style
3. Maximizing one's coping strengths and limiting weaknesses
4. Developing strategies to deal with issues created by disease
5. Exploring the effect of illness on one's sense of self and relationships with others
6. Ventilating feelings and fears
7. Incorporating the present reality of the diagnosis into one's
   sense of past and future

Understanding the Disease

The victim's perceptions of the disease may be far different from a
professional understanding of the disease. The meaning that someone gives to the diagnosis may be inaccurate and may affect him
or her in negative ways. Some people may read the diagnosis as a
death sentence, thereby extinguishing any hope in themselves and
consequently impairing subsequent treatment. Others may take the
diagnosis too lightly, failing to change their life-style or develop
the kinds of behaviors that will enhance health.

One of the first tasks for individuals and families is to try to
understand the disease at issue. This not only means discovering
an accurate and realistic understanding of the disease, but also of
learning to cope in a way that allows continued hope, a sense of
control, and lower levels of anxiety.

This process begins by exploring one's own understanding of the
disease. Often this is best done with a medical professional who
can provide opportunities to probe any misunderstandings and to
gently question misperceptions. During this process it is usually
helpful to explore the sources of one's own information as well as
the validity accorded each source.

It is also important to assess factors that may be blocking one's
own comprehension. In some cases the barriers can be social.

Sometimes one may be intimidated by the social status and authority of the physician or other medical personnel. As a result, one is hesitant to ask questions. There may be educational barriers because of which the ill person has a difficult time understanding the information offered and is reluctant to acknowledge that difficulty. These barriers often reinforce one another. The ill person may not understand the physician's language and may be too embarrassed or intimidated to ask questions.

If this could be a problem, one should ask to have another family member, friend, or some trusted intermediary such as a clergyman present when one hears the results, or at subsequent visits. It may also help to write down any questions that one may have. In that way one can be sure to ask them at the next visit to the physician. Open communication is critical, but it is important to realize, especially in this early period, that not all questions will have definitive answers. Caregivers also should be sensitive enough to present information and to provide access to information in language the person can understand. Offering a trusting, unhurried, respectful, and nonjudgmental context in which people may ask questions, repeating and reviewing what they know, will help this information process. Linking people with other persons of similar backgrounds who have the disease, informally and in self-help groups, is also quite useful. Not only can such information facilitate understanding, it also can offer coping strategies and provide hope. When communication is poor, someone should inform the caregiver.

Caregivers also need to assess the information that a person has. Just because someone lacks formal education does not mean that he or she is unable to understand even highly sophisticated information if his or her life is at stake.

There may be psychological barriers as well. Serious anxiety can make it difficult to absorb and understand information about the disease. One woman told me that she became so nervous once she heard the word "cancer" that she was frozen in fear, unable to hear, respond, or question. Sometimes talking over these fears with others can alleviate anxiety. Or returning at a later time when the level of anxiety has lessened, perhaps supported by a friend, may provide a better opportunity to question and to discuss the illness and its treatment. It also may help to explore the sources of anxiety. Becoming anxious may result from a number of sources: misinformation, prior poor experiences, or a generally pessimistic attitude about life. Negative perceptions due to misinformation or past experiences can generally be handled in the same way as any learning process. In a trusting context, earlier information can be explored, sources evaluated, and new information provided.

It is important to remember that many major life-threatening illnesses lumped together under such categories as "cancer" or "heart disease" are really many different related diseases. An individual's earlier experiences or the experiences of others with cancer or heart disease may tell very little about a similar but different condition. For example, a friend or relative's experience with pancreatic cancer will not be all that relevant for someone who has prostate cancer. Each disease has its own treatment, symptoms, and prognosis. Moreover, the pace of progress of science is not only amazing but constantly accelerating. In 1971 I worked in the pediatric ward of a major cancer center. Most of the children who died of cancer in the past could be successfully treated by today's methods. Even people diagnosed with AIDS today can expect to live considerably longer lives than those diagnosed a decade ago. Again, self-help groups or persons who have the disease may be very useful both in providing the most current information and in reinforcing hope.

Sometimes family members will be worried that the ill individual seems too optimistic. I usually do not find such an optimistic state to be troubling. Overly optimistic perceptions of disease are less problematic at this early stage of illness. Clinicians and researchers have emphasized the value of optimistic orientations toward disease and treatment. Beyond the serious obligation of physicians to provide patients with accurate information about their disease and the risks of treatment, these optimistic perceptions should not be challenged unless they impair adherence with treatment or endanger the lives of others.

Examining and Maximizing Health and Life-Style

Life-threatening illness can often be influenced by one's life-style. In some cases life-style can be a significant contributor to the disease. In other cases life-style factors may have an effect on treatment, course, or reoccurrence of the illness. In any case, good health practices will contribute to reducing stress and facilitating adaptation. Thus it is worthwhile to examine the ways in which one's current life-style affects health, as well as the ways by which one may modify life-style practices to enhance health. Suitable exercises, good nutrition, adequate sleep, and effective stress management are more important when one is seriously ill than ever before. It is important, of course, to discuss any major life-style modification, such as diet or exercise, with one's physician. In addition to improving health, such actions can reaffirm a renewed sense of control over one's life that may have been threatened by the diagnosis.

Maximizing One's Coping Strengths and Limiting Weaknesses

In any crisis—and the diagnosis of life-threatening illness is certainly a crisis—individuals and their families face certain challenges. If they want to focus on the illness in such a way as to maximize chances for successful outcome, they will need to marshal their resources effectively and limit time, energy, and other kinds of losses to problems that might intrude upon this central struggle.

Here again, a good way to begin is by examining one's coping styles and strategies. Often an effective way to start that exploration is to focus on the ways that one has reacted to previous crises in one's life. This method can reveal coping styles and strategies that might be useful now, in this current crisis. For example, if one's previous tendency has been to get angry, such a response in the current crisis should come as no surprise. If in past crises you were prone to make rash decisions or to panic, you may wish to guard against that kind of reaction now.

Focusing on past strategies often helps one to become aware of styles and patterns that may help or hinder current responses. Once one has reviewed past coping strategies, one can consider what strategies can best be adapted to the present crisis. One can also consider which styles work and which styles do not work. For example, anger can be a powerful motivational tool if it focused against the disease. But if anger is directed toward family and friends, that same response may drive people away just at the time when they are most needed. Similarly, if one has a tendency to carefully weigh decisions and is usually reluctant to chose until all the information is in, this characteristic can be helpful in avoiding rash actions. But it can also inhibit fast responses to a crisis. Examining coping styles early in the illness process allows one to draw upon obvious strengths, and also helps one to become aware of weaknesses, perhaps to better overcome them.

I should add that continuity in styles and reactions is not always present. Sometimes we have changed so much that previous ways of coping are no longer indicative of present responses. But sometimes this lack of continuity can be a cause for concern. For example, it might show that the person is in a sustained destructive denial or an immobilizing panic. I always suggest to counselors and other caregivers that if this continuity is absent, they should explore reasons that might account for these new ways of coping.

A second area to consider is social support. Who can one turn to for help? In what ways can the people you know best help? What are one's own feelings about asking for or accepting different kinds of help?

Many times sources of support may be underestimated. Once family and friends are identified and approached, they can surprise one with their willingness to help, each in their own way. During counseling I ask my clients, who can you turn to in crisis? Often they name only a few people, but when I probe deeper, asking them questions about who they have told and who has offered help, they discover that their network is larger than they had realized. In some cases they may recognize that their own inhibitions limit help options. For example, a thirty-year-old man diagnosed with MS was surprised at the help offered by his formerly estranged brother.

When support is not forthcoming, it is often valuble to explore the reasons why. Sometimes possible networks simply do not exist. This is often the case with many elderly people. They may have outlived spouses, family, and friends, or those who remain may be too frail or too ill themselves to offer assistance.

In other cases expectations for help were unrealistic. One client of mine, for example, was outraged that her daughter did not quit her job to care for her. The daughter was more than willing to help when she was not working and to coordinate her mother's care. Her mother's expectations, though, ignored the constraints imposed on her daughter by her own life needs.

Perhaps potential helpers are receiving mixed or ambivalent messages. In one case a man with cancer was annoyed that his adult children did not make themselves more available to help him. Yet whenever they asked what they could do, he put them off. An offer to drive him to the doctor's office would be met by the response, "No thanks, I've called a cab." They felt they were respecting his independence; he believed they should have insisted upon driving. This example indicates the importance of clearly communicating one's needs and desires, and not expecting others to guess what help you need and expect.

Sometimes support may be utilized effectively. I had a professor who said that most people are either listeners or doers. We get into trouble, he would add, when we expect doers to listen and listeners to do. That may be a simplistic notion, but it does emphasize a key point: different people are comfortable helping in different ways. For example, a daughter I know was very uncomfortable with changing her father's medical dressing, but she was happy to cook food for him and to feed him. Another woman became tense when asked to drive her friend to the doctor's office. She deeply wanted to help, but found the particular request painful and often made excuses not to go. After she shared her true feelings she found other ways to help, such as babysitting her friend's children; she thus met her desire to help and fulfilled a real need for her friend. Again, communicating needs to friends and family, and being open about what is helpful and comforting can go a long way toward improving one's support system.

Sometimes one has to recognize that family or friends can be destructive if they encourage negative behaviors such as nonadherence to a regimen or substance abuse. For example, an adolescent with leukemia had a friend who thought the cure for every moment of anxiety or depression was a can of beer. Family and friends whose own needs or behaviors are so extreme that they sap strength rather than providing support do more harm than good. Verbally or physically abusive persons, people whose lives are so chaotic that they constantly involve others in their own crises, or people who are so self-absorbed that even when you are in a crisis they still look to you to meet *their* needs will make your problems worse. Such individuals attack your self-confidence, your self-esteem, your hope. One client coping with his father's cancer told me of a friend with whom he bicycled. The friend would tell constant stories of people he knew who had cancer, often stressing negative outcomes! "For example," this client indicated, "One time when I was discussing my father's chemotherapy, he told a long story about someone's long struggle with chemotherapy. I was waiting for a punchline like 'She's doing well now.' Instead, he told me she died six months later."

There are three ways to deal with other people's destructive behaviors. Some people can just ignore them, attributing that behavior to misguided attempts to help, the destructive individual's own needs and problems, or lack of effective coping abilities. In other cases, it may be necessary to avoid or discontinue a destructive relationship. Or one may have to confront the person, explaining that these behaviors are not helpful and perhaps offering concrete suggestions on how they can help better.

One should not neglect formal sources of support. Many services, including transportation, nursing, home care, support groups, meals, counseling, even financial help, may be available. These can often supplement help from family and friends. Often hospital social workers or agencies such as the American Cancer Society (see Appendix 1) can provide information on what services are available in different communities and how one applies for their help. Finding available help, even as early as the time of the diagnosis when this help may not be necessary, can alleviate anxiety, avoid the difficulties associated with trying to find help at a time when it is critically necessary, and reaffirm one's own abilities to cope.

Part of limiting weaknesses is placing other problems in perspective. It is difficult to cope with the crisis of diagnosis when it is just one of the problems a person is considering. For example, it is doubly devastating to learn that one has AIDS when one is struggling with the psychological crisis of sexual identity. Similarly, an IV drug user, coping with a chaotic life characterized by poverty, addiction, interpersonal problems, and legal difficulties, may simply not have the resources to cope with illness. It is difficult to cope with cancer or heart attack, but more so when the crisis follows divorce or career reverses. In these cases one should prioritize concerns. Focusing on the illness first, and leaving other concerns for later, is one way to avoid being overwhelmed.

Developing Strategies to Deal with Issues Created by Disease

A diagnosis of life-threatening illness creates immediate practical issues that must be resolved. Among the most pressing of these issues are:

Whom to Tell

One needs to make decisions about how much information to reveal and whom to confide in. Given uncertainty about one's fate, one will be very concerned about how much information to share with family and friends, and how that information should be presented. The issue of disclosure is critical for a number of reasons. Among family and friends, disclosure can be an important factor in the ability to mobilize social support throughout the course of illness. If you keep a diagnosis secret, your intimates may be deprived of opportunities to share information and offer support. One friend told me an illustrative story. He had made an appointment for tests but decided not to share this news with his brother and sister, for he did not wish to upset them. For a week he and his wife struggled with their anxiety. At his physician's office he learned that the condition was minor and easily treated. When he shared his joy at this news with his siblings, they told him they both had the same problem. Had he shared news about his health problem earlier, he and his wife would have been spared an anxious week. Disclosing news about disease to others can be a positive experience. Many ill people find that family and friends are far more supportive and helpful than they had expected. Disclosure allows others to show concern and offer support.

Sometimes the issue of disclosure or how much to communicate comes up just in deciding how to answer the question "How are you?" A colleague with leukemia struggled with the problem of how to respond to this common question and finally decided to respond, "I'm doing very well, thank you, though I do have a serious disease."

Sometimes individuals find it useful to rehearse ways to disclose the disease with a confidante. Others ask a family member or confidante to share news about the diagnosis with other family and friends. As one woman explained, "It got us past the 'awkward moment' and it allowed friends to respond as they wanted. Most called and were very supportive."

While friends and family generally are supportive, it often takes a little time for relationships to return to normalcy. One woman mentioned that it took her friends about two weeks before they would talk about their own problems again.

People diagnosed with a serious disease may be very secretive about their problems for a number of reasons. They may not have come to terms with the diagnosis themselves. Secretiveness can be a form of control; if an individual feels that he or she cannot control the disease, the individual might take some comfort from knowing that he or she can control who else knows and what they know. One adolescent diagnosed with leukemia, for example, swore school officials to secrecy. She later told her classmates the diagnosis, in turn swearing each one to secrecy. Some people may wish to protect others or they may wish to protect themselves. They may be anxious, perhaps realistically so, that disclosure will affect their relationships with others, their plans, and their careers. The pressure to keep things secret is particularly strong whenever the disease is highly stigmatizing, as with AIDS.

Ill individuals need to remember that attempts to jealously guard information can be counterproductive. Family and friends can often sense an intimate's anxiety. Coworkers will attempt to make sense of frequent absences, changes in behavior, and changes in appearance. Given the relative medical sophistication of many people in our society, they will evaluate the information they receive from the evidence they observe. Inconsistent accounts made to different individuals can create confusion and rumors. Insurance claims, visits to medical personnel, and other such factors may yield significant clues to the diagnosis. In short, one's ability to actually control information is probably quite limited— especially as time goes on. Secretiveness may backfire, for rumors about the diagnosis can often be far more damaging than the truth. Moreover, excessive secretiveness can harm relationships by undermining trust.

It is important to remember that disclosure decisions do not have to be put in all or nothing terms. Decisions need not be cast in the form, "Whom do I choose to tell or not to tell?" Instead, the question can be posed as, "What information do I need to share with which others, at what point?"

Coping with Medical Professionals

One may need assistance in coping with medical professionals. During the diagnostic phase many people have many important concerns about what course of action to pursue. Should they seek a second opinion? Are they comfortable with their physicians and specialists? If further testing or exploratory surgery is contemplated, are they satisfied with the medical facility?

Feelings about professionals need to be explored. In some cases discomfort or ambivalence may be a result of anxiety over the diagnosis or anger at a physician for delivering bad news. But in other cases ambivalence or discomfort may reflect realistic concerns. Not every physician is the perfect physician for you, nor is every hospital or specialized medical facility equally good for you as a place of treatment.

While reviewing these feelings, it helps to remember that a second opinion may be a good idea; another doctor may well offer valuable medical advice and alternatives for treatment. He or she may cushion the shock of diagnosis, return a sense of control, and even provide a sense of valuable space and time to make critical decisions. But second opinions can be a problem if they delay treatment beyond a time that is medically wise or if they lead to "shopping around" for third, fourth, or fifth opinions, deferring the reality of the diagnosis and a reasoned course of treatment.

It is important for individuals and their families to be comfortable with both their physicians and their hospital. This became clear when my father was diagnosed with cancer. While we had great respect for his physician, we were not comfortable with the local general hospital that was handling father's operation. As a family we decided that it would be best if father were treated at a major medical center even if such treatment meant switching to another physician. My father's physician was understanding and supportive of my father's and our family's decision. Although we did not wish to hurt the doctor's feelings, my father's health was our first priority. The situation was successfully resolved. My father recovered from the surgery. But even if the ending had not been so happy, insisting that our father be treated in a more sophisticated medical facility was the right thing for us to do. Had he died, at least we would have known that we had done all we could to make sure he had the best possible care.

Deciding on Treatments

After a diagnosis of life-threatening disease, individuals will need to make decisions about treatment. Treatment plans differ according to the illness involved. In some cases, treatment plans may be relatively unobtrusive. Some conditions require little more than monitoring. With others, medication or life-style modifications may be recommended. When a friend had a heart attack, for example, his doctors prescribed medication, placed him on a diet, and recommended that he review and simplify his life-style, eliminating unnecessary stress.

With many conditions, though, other approaches are necessary. In many cases surgery, radiation therapy, or chemotherapy will be required. Whatever therapies are available, individuals should explore their feelings and fears about them. An individual may fear surgery because she fears anesthesia, loss of consciousness, postoperative pain, visible damage (scars and the like), loss of function, aftereffects on employment and finances, or any combination of these things. Radiation may be feared because of the procedure itself (treatment from a machine with no human present), concerns over side effects such as sexual dysfunction and/or sterility, or effects on later health. Chemotherapy can engender similar fears. In all these cases individuals may be afraid that the cure will be worse than the illness.

It is important that one discusses and shares such fears with physicians. Sometimes these fears may be based upon past experiences that are no longer valid, or perhaps not relevant in this case. One might be needlessly troubled, or worse, even refuse lifesaving therapy because of baseless misperceptions.

It is also critical to discuss other options and choices that might be available. Again, second opinions may prove valuable. I also strongly believe that people who are very active participants in health decisions, who maintain a strong sense of control rather than simply passively accepting a physician's advice, who actively research and discuss treatment options, are not only likely to cope better, but may, in fact, live longer.

One may also need to carefully consider risks and side effects. Physicians are usually very careful about outlining *all* the possible things that *could* happen as a result of therapy. Physicians are morally and legally required to inform one of risks. Not everyone will experience side effects in the same way. Siegal (1986) emphasizes the importance of positive thinking. He believes that if one focuses on all the bad things that can or might happen, this can be self-fulfilling. Seigal recommends that one develop mental attitudes that stress minimal discomfort. Seigal also teaches positive ways to envision therapies, for example, imagining radiation as a warm, golden beam of healing light.

These treatment decisions can often be confused by the fact that one is getting contrary advice on treatment from physicians and others. It is important to examine any conflicting advice with a physician you trust or perhaps with a counselor. Sometimes these conflicts are more apparent than real. For example, some unconventional holistic therapies such as diets or imaging work well in conjunction with conventional medical therapies.

At other times, though, there are medical disagreements about what is the best way to proceed. Here counselors can help you to find the information you need to make an intelligent decision. Information from physicians about possible risks and benefits will be essential. Counselors can sometimes suggest options that can be discussed with physicians. For example, perhaps there is time to try less-radical approaches, leaving more-radical alternatives for later stages of treatment, if needed. It is critical to spend time examining these choices, even given the anxiety often felt in this period and the pressure to make a decision quickly. If one has fully explored one's options, one is less likely to second guess or regret these decisions later.

It is also important to know how treatment might affect other aspects of life. Often if potential problems are identified, compromises may be found that might alleviate some concerns. For example, if someone is concerned that therapy might impair work or school, it might be scheduled on a Friday or just before a long holiday weekend so that side effects have subsided by the beginning of the next work or school week.

In addition to conventional therapies, one might also consider unconventional treatments. It might be a good idea to explore approaches that seek to enhance the immune-system functioning by means of diet, exercise, physical therapies, imaging, positive thinking, or even forms of faith healing. When my father was ill with cancer, my gift to him was teaching him imaging. Imaging means utilizing a person's imagination in a very active way. Its underlying assumption is that there are strong associations between mental and physical states, and mental attitude may be able to enhance the functioning of the immune system. In my father's case, we developed images that were familiar and comfortable to him. He imagined his immune cells as soldiers seeking out and destroying enemy cancer cells. Each day he set aside time to develop this mental image of a large but successful battle.

In recent years a great deal of attention has been given to holistic and unconventional therapies. My own view is that when these treatments are used as compliments to conventional medical treatment, do not discourage medical treatment, and carry no medical risk, interest and involvement should be encouraged. Complimentary therapies such as imaging, positive thinking, and therapeutic uses of humor and touch (to name a few), may allow one to gain a renewed sense of control over one's illness and may enhance coping. Since we really do not fully understand the unique blend of physiological, medical, psychological, and social factors that influence the course of an illness in any particular individual, caregivers should not discourage individuals from availing themselves of alternate therapies when they enhance hope.

If one does make a decision to seek an alternative method of treatment *instead of* a more-traditional approach, it is important to understand and evaluate that choice. Sometimes it may result from social pressures such as advice from family or friends. Sometimes such approaches may result from feelings of helplessness or panic that move one to seek treatment, however unproven, that seems to offer more than traditional medicine. Sometimes finding a physician who provides emotional support and allows one to clearly review all treatment options may mitigate a desire to attempt unconventional approaches. And if one still chooses to go this route, it is important to have a physician who is understandong should one later decide to seek more-traditional treatment.

Other Life Choices

The diagnosis of life-threatening illness may also force decisions in other areas of life: "Should I proceed with the wedding?" "Should I pursue this relationship?" "Should I quit school or work?" These examples illustrate the kind of questions one may feel a need to consider.

There are two contrasting coping tendencies. One is to keep things exactly the same, proceeding with life as if there were no existing crisis. This approach is unlikely to work, because disease already has created or soon will create changes that must be confronted. Pretending that they do not exist impairs the kind of realistic planning that may allow a renewed sense of control. While one cannot control the fact that a diagnosis has changed one's life, to some extent one can control *the way* it changes life. One client of mine provides a good illustration of this important point. Insisting that his diagnosis changed nothing, he worked as hard or even harder in his small business. But when he was hospitalized as a result of exhaustion, he finally had to admit that his diagnosis had changed his life. Now he was now able to realistically plan his workday. He limited himself to about four hours a day, regulated the tasks he did, and hired additional help. His new plan allowed him to marshall his resources and cope more effectively with his health crisis. When he recognized that he could still make good decisions, even in the midst of a crisis, he regained a sense of his own coping abilities.

Others may week to make definitive decisions regarding all possible contingencies, often ignoring the inherent uncertainty of this phase of their lives. Sometimes it is better to wait, prioritizing issues that need to be settled now and leaving others for a later time. It is important to recognize that similar decisions can have very distinct meanings and implications to different individuals, or at different times in the illness. The decision to quit work can represent a premature and unhealthy withdrawal or a life-enhancing decision about priorities. It may profoundly affect financial stability by limiting income, access to health insurance, and the availability of other forms of help. Given the uncertainty of this phase, it is often worthwhile to remember that decisions can be tentative and limited. Instead of asking oneself, "Should I quit work?," one might better focus on more limited possibilities, such as taking a temporary leave of absence, scaling back commitments and work, a shorter day or week, or even working at home. Review and discuss these decisions with all those who may be affected by them.

Finally, one may want to consider other contingencies. This may be a good time to review your will or to make one if you don't have one, and to consider issues of guardianship, health proxies, power of attorney, living wills, and the like. Health proxies allow another to make treatment decisions if one is no longer able to do so. Power of attorney is a document that allows someone else to legally make decisions for you when you are no longer competent to do so. "Living wills" are documents that express a desire not to have extraordinary means used to preserve life when death is inevitable. While they are legally binding only in some states, they are helpful as an expression of the individual's wishes that may facilitate both the family's and the physician's decisions. It is always worthwhile to periodically review titles, leases, wills, and insurance policies to see if decisions on property, beneficiaries, guardians, and executors reflect current relationships. An illness is simply one more opportunity to reexamine these earlier decisions.

Exploring the Effect of Illness on Sense of Self and Relationships with Others

The diagnosis of life-threatening illness changes one's sense of self in many ways. One may feel betrayed by the frailty of one's physical body. One may feel stigmatized by disease. Critical identities may seem threatened by the illness: a teacher may be anxious that he or she will no longer be able to teach, an avid skier may fear the end of that activity. It is important to discuss these concerns with caregivers, especially physicians and counselors, and to raise them in self-help groups. This may provide opportunities to ventilate these feelings, find reassurance, and sometimes develop new strategies to deal with the problem. One fifty-five-year-old man facing a colostomy was worried that the operation, if he chose to have it, would effectively end his career. He discussed this concern with his physician, who recommended a support group. In the support group he found reassurance that his fears were natural but groundless.

A life-threatening illness is likely to change relationships with other people. They may not know how to respond, especially in the early phase of illness, to the newly diagnosed person, perhaps someone who is in the paradoxical position of looking well and yet being seriously ill. Some friends or family may feel awkward and uneasy, anxious about the disease, fearful of how it may change the relationship, unsure of how to act or what to say. Feeling such discomfort, they may very well avoid both the ill individual and even other family members.

If one is feeling disappointed by the reactions of others, it is usually worthwhile to explore this issue early, for often these things can escalate later on in the illness. That is, later on people may be avoiding you in part because they feel guilty about their previous avoidance! Exploring these feelings with counselors or other caregivers may provide opportunities not only to ventilate these concerns, but also to develop strategies for dealing with change. Sometimes humor can break the ice. At other times it may be worthwhile to gently confront the issue. One friend diagnosed with leukemia had to confront his fishing buddies. They admitted that they had had extended conversations among themselves as to whether he was well enough to be invited on a trip. He needed to gently remind them that he could make that decision himself, but first they would have to invite him. Life-threatening illness can bring isolation or greater intimacy. What actually happens is the responsibility of everyone: the ill person, family, and friends.

Ventilating Feelings and Fears

At any phase of illness one may experience strong emotional reactions. Individuals and families may have all types of feelings ranging from relief that the uncertainty "is over" to deep depression at the results. Almost any emotions may be experienced throughout the course of illness. There is no one set of normal reactions, nor any one sequence of emotional experiences. Each person will respond in his or her own individual ways.

Dealing with emotional reactions can be difficult. Often people experiencing illness face a double bind. They are filled with feelings, but may find limited opportunities to share them. There can be many reasons for this situation. They may be reluctant to share their feelings and their fears, especially with those whom they most love. Or family and friends may find it difficult to listen. Family and friends may deny the sick individual's negative feelings, telling him or her not to feel angry, guilty, or sad—as if such feelings can be so readily dismissed.

Often self-help groups or counselors can provide the emotional distance and objectivity that people need if they are to ventilate their true feelings. Three things are essential: understanding one's feelings, and expressing them, and using them constructively in the course of the illness.

Individuals experiencing life-threatening illness need opportunities to talk over their concerns in a trusting, nonjudgmental atmosphere. Once these feelings are openly expressed, an individual can move on to explore both the sources of these emotions and the ways that this affect will influence treatment.

Caregivers should try to assist individuals in utilizing feelings constructively in the subsequent treatment of illness. For example, emotions such as fear and guilt can immobilize or motivate. Anger can isolate one from others, imperiling relationships, or it can be focused against the disease.

A case illustrates the ways that individuals can deal with their feelings and fears. A thirty-year-old male homosexual was diagnosed as HIV positive. He initially responded with a fear of future pain and suffering, and with guilt that his present pain was punishment for his life-style. In counseling he was able both to express these concerns and to explore his fear and guilt. Honest, realistic communication with his physician alleviated his anxiety somewhat. He recognized the uncertain course of the disease, but was reassured by his physician that the doctor would do everything possible to minimize pain. Instruction in self-hypnosis and imaging gave him some sense of control over possible future pain. He was also able to explore his guilt. He recognized that this guilt reflected ambivalent feelings about his sexual identity, an issue he thought he had resolved. He was able to understand factors that contributed to that ambivalence. Accepting his homosexuality, he was also able to affirm that within his identity he still retained choices. He was able to regret some of his past choices, particularly relating to promiscuous, anonymous sex. But while recognizing his past actions as a factor in infection, he was able to understand his behavior in the context of the time. Exploring his own religious beliefs, he could also reject a belief in a punishing God. And he was able to affirm that he could use his choices to avoid spreading the virus, minimize future exposure, and maximize health.

One should recognize that any and each emotional reaction can have both constructive and destructive manifestations. As an individual expresses and explores his or her feelings, he or she is able to minimize destructive aspects and facilitate effective responses toward the illness.

Incorporating the Present Reality of the Diagnosis into One's Sense of Past and Future

The diagnosis of illness affects not only the present but one's past and future. The very nature of dealing with life-threatening issues may compel one to focus on past issues. Previous ways of coping with crisis, expectations of support, and experiences with illness are topics that involve considerable history. They bring one back to unresolved issues, perhaps dealing with dependency, sexuality, or relationships, that are now reactivated by the diagnosis. One may wish to discuss these reemerging issues with counselors and therapists, particularly if they seem to be interfering with the way one currently is functioning. For example, Louis, a twenty-five-year-old man, newly diagnosed with muscular dystrophy, found that he needed to work through his fears of abandonment. Louis had been placed in foster care when his mother could not cope with his ill brother. Based on this early experience, Louis feared that his wife would abandon him too. His fears and his constant demands for reassurance actually threatened his marriage. Through therapy, he was able to understand the source of his fears and work on resolving these early issues.

The diagnosis of life-threatening illness also calls one's future life into question. Not only health, but all facets of the previous life-style, such as priorities and relationships, are opened to review. Many individuals who recover from illness often speak of the diagnosis as a positive and pivotal turning point in their lives. The illness provided an opportunity, however unwelcome and unsought, to review and to change their lives. In one case, a woman who had been a workaholic reprioritized her time so that she could spend more time in leisure activities with her children and her friends.

Even when recovery is not expected, one can decide how one wishes to spend the time that one has left. A recent study of persons with AIDS found that many individuals made decisions to reprioritize time and activities, spending more time with family and friends. Not only does this affirm personal control but it also may alleviate anxiety, bolster social support, and provide useful diversion, making remaining time more enjoyable and meaningful.

I firmly believe that the ability to see past the crisis, to seize the opportunity, to make changes, is a critical factor in maintaining a positive attitude. Regardless of the circumstances, strive to continue the plan. Seek stimulation. The same human needs that existed prior to the crisis still exist now. Continue to plan for the future, even if decisions are constrained by a more-limited time frame. Planning provides a sense of diversion and reinforces hope. For example, one man with cancer researched and planned the cruise he and his wife intended to take when he recovered. And he lived to take that cruise. Looking beyond the illness, resetting priorities, and reviewing what you want from life not only improves the present quality of life, it also enhances survival.

The End of the Acute Phase

The acute phase of life-threatening illness, centering on diagnosis, is by its very nature self-limiting. For though it may take a period of time, perhaps weeks, the uncertainty of the acute phase will be at least partially resolved and individuals and their families will face new realities. These realities can differ. In rare situations the event precipitating the diagnosis may result in death or a swift decline into the terminal phase of illness. Here loss may be sudden as with a fatal heart attack or death on the operating table. This leaves survivors to deal with diagnosis and death almost simultaneously. Or the illness may progress so rapidly, or the disability, perhaps from stroke, be so pronounced and irreversible that the individual and family have to grieve the extensive losses that have occurred and prepare for the person's likely death.

Then there are situations in which recovery is considered complete. Here the person may have recovered from a heart attack or stroke or have been successfully treated for cancer. In these situations, people may face varied risks of recurrence. However, even with recovery, there still seems to be considerable aftereffects from an encounter with life-threatening illness. Koocher and O'Malley (1981) studied almost 120 survivors of childhood cancer. They found that these people still suffered from varied residues of the disease including physical scars, fears of relapse, psychological impairment, and discrimination in employment as well as in obtaining health and life insurance. Even full recovery may leave physical, emotional, psychological, social, and financial scars that may reverberate throughout one's life.

In many cases, though, individuals and their families will have to cope with the ongoing presence of disease, its treatment, and consequent levels of disability. Here the person enters the chronic phase of illness, a phase with its own challenges and tasks.

5

Living with Disease

The Chronic Phase: An Overview

It is a tedious time of testing and treatment. There are bi-monthly chemotherapy sessions, which leave Joan, a fifty-four-year-old cancer patient, sick and exhausted for days. In between those times Joan cares for her home and maintains her position as an elementary-school guidance counselor. Her latest prognosis is guarded but optimistic. Within six months the chemotherapy will end. But it will be five years, perhaps longer, before she knows, with only reasonable certainty, whether she will survive this bout with cancer. Meanwhile her days are filled with a low level of continued stress punctuated by occasional waves of anxiety. Her nights are times of fitful sleep and troubled dreams.

Joan's experience is an increasingly common one in life-threatening illness. Most people will neither quickly recover from the disease nor rapidly deteriorate. For most, between the diagnosis and the outcome of the disease, there will be a long chronic period during which one struggles with the demands and side effects of treatment, the symptoms of the disease, and the daily business of living. Weisman (1980), in his study of responses to cancer, described the early part of this chronic phase as "accommodation and mitigation." For Weisman, the challenge of this period is to accommodate the illness with previous coping skills and roles. Often by this time the crisis posed by the diagnosis is mitigated. The ill individual is simply striving now to find ways to live life with the ongoing presence of the disease.

Perhaps the most dramatic change in life-threatening illness is the existence and extension of the chronic phase. Not too many years ago the period between diagnosis and death for many illnesses was typically measured in months, and these months were mostly lived within hospital walls. Now that period may be measured in years, allowing hope for a still-undiscovered cure or ongoing remission, and much of it may be lived in the person's own environment, permitting the resumption of work, school, and other roles.

AIDS provides a good illustration of this important point. Persons diagnosed with AIDS may live a number of years. Throughout this time they may harbor hopes, hardly unrealistic, that newly developed treatments will continue to extend life or even cure the disease. They may work or go to school, as well as continue to develop relationships. There may be long periods when symptoms seem under control and health seems good. Though the disease is present and likely to shorten life, the individual continues to live.

This new reality of life-threatening illness has blurred the distinction between chronic and life-threatening illness. The chronic phase of life-threatening illness can be defined as that period between diagnosis and the final outcome. Here the person attempts to cope with the demands of life while simultaneously striving to maintain health and prevent and/or adapt to the deterioration of health caused by the presence of life-threatening disease. The chronic phase involves many of the same issues and struggles common to all chronic illness.

The quality of life in the chronic phase is likely to be deeply affected by the nature and symptoms of the disease. While these two factors were explored earlier, they deserve mention here again.

The trajectory or pattern that the illness takes often shapes the experience of the chronic phase. In diseases that show a slow but steady or relentless pattern of decline, individuals and their families may have to cope with the psychological distress of constant and continued deterioration. "Every night," one young muscular dystrophy victim told me, "I go to bed knowing I will wake up weaker." In these patterns there may be a sense of great weariness, of having lived too long. To capture her mood, one client once paraphrased the words of the Indian leader Chief Joseph when he surrendered to U.S. forces: "I have fought too long forever." Not only are these slow periods of decline difficult for ill individuals, they are difficult for their families and others involved with the person as well.

Other patterns or trajectories may shape this experience in other ways. Patterns marked by relapses and remissions as well as those where periods of relative stability are followed by sharp declines create their own unique problems for ill individuals and their families. Relapses are times of great anxiety. One woman with MS said, "I never know with each relapse how far I will decline, how disabled I will come, how dependent.p . . . and I always think 'Will I be able to recover? Will I have to enter the nursing home?' "A man with AIDS, a disease characterized by remission and relapse rather than the declining plateaus of MS, echoed her concern: "Each relapse I say 'How long [to live]' and with each remission I ask the same question." And both noted the effects of the illness on other aspects of life. The person with AIDS, for example, described how hard it was to plan, to readjust, and even to relate to friends and family. "I have had," he once dramatically announced "more deathbed scenes than Sarah Bernhardt." In each illness, though, the nature of the trajectory will define the types of difficulties and experiences individuals encounter.

The quality of life in this chronic phase also will be greatly affected and defined by the particular symptoms of the underlying disease. In situations where one is asymptomatic or experiences minor symptoms and little pain, it may be possible to continue to maintain a good quality of life, one that approaches the standard of life prior to the diagnosis. In other cases, where symptoms are persistent, recurring, and disruptive, and pain is chronic, the quality of life may be disrupted. Regardless of the level of disruption it is natural that many individuals and their families can be affected by chronic anxiety.

In the early phases of the disease, or in periods of remission, the nature of life may not change dramatically from earlier, preillness times. Often this is very reassuring to individuals and families, a reminder that a good quality of life can be maintained even in the face of life-threatening illness. Hope may reassert itself. Individuals may become busy in treatment and even engage and explore alternate modalities of treatment such as imaging or other attitudinal approaches.

Some individuals may also use this time to plan for the possible events and contingencies likely to occur as the illness progresses. Illness often compels individuals to make financial arrangements and to address other pressing concerns such as childcare. People may need to anticipate medical and care needs and allocate and prioritize time. This planning may mitigate some of the loss of control experienced at the time of diagnosis. It is important to remember, though, that some individuals and family members may approach this in a different way, preferring to take each day one at a time.

Life in the chronic phase is often punctuated by varied crisis points. Crisis points can include the complications, deteriorations, and relapses brought on by the illness, as well as the side effects and complications of treatments. Even unrelated and minor illnesses can create crises. For example, the symptoms of a common cold can cause consternation either as a threat to the precarious balance between health and illness or as a harbinger of death, causing anxiety that this simple symptom evidences a final decline.

To others, increasing dependency and perhaps even life events can create psychological distress and crisis. To a young man with muscular dystrophy, the dependency symbolized by a wheel chair can be profoundly distressing. In another case, a man with cancer was devastated when he learned he would be moved from an acute-care institution to a chronic facility instead of going home. This placement reinforced his perception of his deterioration and increased dependency. It reminded him that remissions would no longer be total and that preserving normalcy would be increasingly difficult.

While the chronic phase can be a difficult period, it can also be perceived as a time of opportunities. The chronic phase often provides opportunities to return to work or school. It can be an opportunity to resume or renew relationships. It can even be an opportunity to fulfill a previously unfulfilled dream. Living with disease is always a difficult, unwanted challenge. But it is a challenge that can be met if one emphasizes that one is *living* with disease.

The chronic phase can be viewed as a transitional and uncertain phase. Throughout this period individuals and families experience significant changes and challenges. Individuals have to confront a series of tasks that reflect that struggle:

1. Managing symptoms and side effects
2. Carrying out medical regimens
3. Preventing and managing medical crises
4. Managing stress and examining coping
5. Maximizing social support and minimizing social isolation
6. Normalizing life in the face of disease
7. Dealing with financial concerns
8. Preserving self-concept
9. Redefining relationships with others throughout the course of the disease
10. Ventilating feelings and fears
11. Finding meaning in suffering, chronicity, uncertainty, or decline

Managing Symptoms and Side Effects

Throughout the chronic phase individuals must constantly cope with the presence of disruptive symptoms and treatment side effects. Often the most intrusive of these is the presence of pain. In the chronic phase pain control is particularly critical since it can discourage adherence to a needed regimen, disrupt other roles, and impair psychological functioning and morale. But while pain control is critical in the chronic phase, it can often be difficult. Pain may be an unavoidable side effect of life-sustaining treatments. It may provide an early warning of crisis, a function that might be lost if one is too medicated. And the possibility of addiction and the effect of pain-control medication on health cannot be ignored even in the chronic phase.

The first step in pain control is always an assessment of both pain and the behavior that results from the pain. Pain is quite complex, more than simply a physical sensation. One needs to assess the ways that pain is influenced by psychological states, spiritual concerns, or social factors. For example, pain can be exacerbated by anxiety or depression. Stress can affect the perception of pain. Even social factors can play a role. Some families may act to reinforce either "pain" or "well" behaviors, perhaps by only responding to the individual's complaints. Often, assessing the patterns of pain (for example, when does pain most often occur) can be a good way to determine influencing factors. For example, in one case one man experienced most severe pain on weekends. Two contributing factors emerged upon analysis. First, the pain preceded chemotherapy always scheduled on Monday, suggesting that anxiety over treatment contributed to pain. Second, other family members were available and solicitous on weekends, suggesting that they too often reinforced pain behaviors by their constant inquiries, sympathy, and solicitous attention.

Once an assessment is made, the caregiver can work with families and others in developing pain-control strategies. In some cases medication will be called for, but medication is likely to be only one strategy in an overall plan of care. Counseling may be a useful strategy as well, allowing one to address underlying psychological, spiritual, or social factors. Both individuals and their families may need to learn principles of positive reinforcement so that "well" behaviors rather than "pain" behaviors can be activated and utilized. Diversion, relaxation techniques, and hypnosis are other possible additional strategies. Even exercise may be useful since it provides diversion, loosens muscle tightness, and reaffirms activity and control.

One very successful strategy that can be employed is imagery. Here one utilizes one's own imaginative processes to alleviate pain. Imagery begins similarly to relaxation techniques. One sits quietly in a comfortable position with closed eyes. Slowly and deeply breathing through the nose, one attempts to relax all muscles, often starting at the feet and moving to the face. When one is relaxed, one is guided to utilize imagination. In some cases the image evoked is a pleasant diversion. For example, one can select and imagine oneself beside a mountain stream or on a Caribbean island. Naturally, such images are drawn from one's own experiences and fantasies. In other cases the person may imagine a healing presence that removes the pain, perhaps, for example, a religious figure. Other forms of imaging may involve conceptualizing the pain on a scale, then imagining the scale value declining as the pain moderates.

There are two points that one should remember. First, effective pain control will often involve a series of strategies. Second, these strategies will have to be customized to the individual. Religious images may be a very useful technique for some, but for others such images would convey little meaning.

While pain may be a significant factor, it is not the only symptom with which individuals may have to cope. There may be a series of side effects and symptoms that one may encounter.

If one is experiencing any symptoms or side effects, it is important to share information about them with one's physician immediately. Often one may be reluctant to do this, not wanting to appear to be a complainer, or because one mistakenly assumes that the problem is part of the illness. Physicians can frequently use this information to better understand your condition and to guide treatment. Many times physicians may be able to take steps to alleviate side effects. Many side effects of treatment or symptoms of diseases can be mitigated by patients' actions or controlled by medication. For example, nausea and vomiting may be lessened by changes in diet, environment, or activity. Medications can also assist. If you discuss such experiences with your physicians, they may be able to suggest some techniques or prescribe some medications that might be helpful. Often individuals will have to experiment with a number of approaches before they find what works best for them. It is especially important not to take any nonprescribed drugs, even over-the-counter drugs, without discussing it with a physician. Even when your physicians are unable to mitigate the symptom, they might at least be able to reassure you that the symptom is expected and not necessarily a sign that the disease is progressing.

When it is not possible to mitigate symptoms, one must try to understand the ways in which these symptoms are affecting one's life. In some cases symptoms may be minimal and easily hidden, but in other cases they may be very apparent and highly disruptive. Individuals may not only experience the disruptive effects of the symptoms on their other roles, but may also feel a sense of stigma that deeply affects not only their own sense of identity and self-esteem but their interaction with others. To cite an example, I know a young man who was disfigured by facial lesions. He felt so stigmatized by these lesions that he hid himself in this apartment, avoiding the visits and social support of friends and family.

One also should review whether any factors in one's life-style, such as activity, distress, or diet, exacerbate stress. Once all of these factors are understood, one can begin to solve any problems about the effects of these symptoms.

In some cases this may involve simple behavioral modification. Anselm Strauss (1975), for example, in his study of chronic illness, describes how an individual experiencing diarrhea had to find stores that permitted easy access to rest rooms. In other cases life-style modifications may be more intensive. One client of mine learned to schedule important meetings prior to lunch since he tired later in the day.

One may need to make environmental modifications as well. One man with limited mobility due to his disease found it necessary to modify his home environment so that he could function on one floor. Sometimes such modifications may involve the cooperation of others. One young boy suffering from leukemia underwent chemotherapy every Friday afternoon. Usually he wasn't functioning well until Tuesday. On Fridays he was so anxious that he found it hard to concentrate on school work. His teacher was extremely helpful with this problem, for she scheduled significant tests and assignments on Wednesdays and Thursdays. Once symptoms and their consequences are explored, often one can work to control them.

Carrying Out Health Regimens

One of the most critical tasks in the chronic phase is carrying out a medical regimen since such regimens are a significant factor in whether a cure or a significant prolongation of life can be achieved. Regimes may range from heavy treatment, such as weekly chemotherapy, or massive changes in life-style and diet that adversely effect the quality of life, to minor life-style changes and simple monitoring. In most cases individuals have to undergo some treatment and adhere to a medical regimen that is itself an intrusion into daily life and a constant reminder of illness. Recently many caregivers have begun to speak of "adherence" to a medical regimen rather than the traditional term "compliance"; adherence emphasizes the sense of partnership so critical to success, rather than simply following a prescribed set of rules provided by caregivers.

Adherence can be difficult for many people, but certain groups have special problems. Adolescents may find treatment restrictions not only burdensome but a threat to their emerging independence and quest for social acceptance. In addition to these types of psychosocial barriers, there may be situational barriers as well. People experiencing too many crises or operating under severe constraints may find adherence difficult. Persons with limited incomes, for example, may find the costs of special diets prohibitive. Others may find instructions and directions confusing. And those with chaotic life-styles characterized by constant crises, such as IV drug users, may find compliance virtually impossible. People who are experiencing multiple chronic illnesses may find it difficult to balance the demands of many simultaneous regimens.

While adherence may be more difficult in these situations, studies (Lubkin, 1986) suggest that almost a third of all individuals do not fully adhere to the treatment regimen. Individuals, families, physicians, and other caregivers must therefore create a partnership to help make adherence work.

This partnership begins when individuals clearly identify and discuss their fears and beliefs about the regimen with their physicians. Often, one significant psychological barrier to adherence is the belief that action will have little effect on the disease. Since this belief will lessen the motivation for adherence, it can become self-fulfilling. A regimen half-followed is unlikely to be successful. Physicians can help by being realistic and truthful about goals, side effects, costs, and expectations. If an individual is told the truth, for example, that symptom relief may be partial, that pain will decrease though not disappear, or that the disease will be slowed but not eradicated, he or she will have realistic expectations and therefore be more likely to follow the regimen. When one recognizes the regimen is doing what is expected, one is more likely to continue to adhere to it.

Tailoring regimens also means fitting them as much as possible into an individual's life-style. Physicians can sometimes make arbitrary decisions on when medication is to be taken without ever discussing how the regimen fits into a person's life. Sometimes issues are minor. One elderly friend had to take medication three times a day. The physician wrote on the prescription "Take at 8 A.M., 4 P.M., 12 A.M." This caused some conflict: my friend was generally asleep by midnight, and at 8 A.M. he was out of his house on a brisk walk. He was reluctant to call his doctor and unsure that he should arbitrarily change the times, but a brief phone call solved his problem: the doctor altered the times for medication to 7 A.M., 3 P.M., 11 P.M. In another situation a client did not take medication because it made her groggy and interfered with her work. When she discussed this problem with her physician, he shifted medication time to the afternoon. My client learned to adjust her work around it. Both cases were readily solved, yet both sets of difficulties, however minor, could have been avoided if physicians and their patients simply talked with one another. Personalizing regimens is usually not difficult, but it does require a level of communication between physicians and their patients that allows for fitting treatment needs to the individual's life-style.

The partnership, though, goes beyond an individual and his or her physicians. Sometimes it involves other caregivers such as nurses. They too may need to be involved in training and educating individuals about their regimens. Often individuals will need ongoing support. For example, one visiting nurse was extraordinarily helpful to an older man who was taking triweekly shots of Interferon. He was expected to inject himself and this made him very anxious. His nurse was very reassuring, constantly showing him the technique, and promising that she would be there as long as he needed her. Even after he mastered injecting himself, she would call periodically to monitor his success and reassure him. Such continuity, empathy, support, and communication between individuals and their caregivers can facilitates adherence to a regimen.

The partnership may also involve family. Sometimes persons within an individual's circle who are discouraging adherence. In one case, for example, whenever Rita was undergoing radiation therapy, an aunt would wonder aloud whether it was worth it. In another case, Tom, a young man undergoing chemotherapy, was often encouraged to drink by a friend, despite the fact that Tom had indicated that drinking interfered with his treatment. In such cases it is important to identify destructive individuals and develop effective strategies for dealing with them. In the first case, Rita was able to share her feelings with her aunt. In the second, Tom found he could not continue what he realized was a destructive relationship.

In some cases family members may be expected to participate in the regimen, but they may be untrained, find their role emotionally or physically difficult, or simply have overwhelming demands on time. They too may need training and perhaps counseling and support to fulfill a new role as caregivers.

One's level of adherence is unlikely to be stable. It is important to review constantly what factors may be facilitating or limiting adherence. Sometimes it may be medical, for example, individuals can feel very discouraged after a crisis or continued deterioration. Sometimes it is psychological: when people are feeling very bad, or even perhaps very good, they may find it difficult to adhere. Sometimes there are other reasons. Perhaps adherence declined in time of high stress or activity. Changes in the social environment may affect adherence. For example, the death of a spouse may influence the surviving spouse's adherence. In one case the husband supervised his wife's medication. When he died, her adherence became much less regular.

Again, partnership means that one should continue to discuss problems as they arise with physicians and caregivers. Identifying barriers to full adherence is often the first step to finding ways to address them. One divorced man struggling with cancer found that his adherence declined when his children visited. He was so involved with them that he often forgot his medication. Once he identified the problem, he and his nurse set up a pill box and a set of alarm clocks.

It is also important not to become discouraged if one finds it difficult to adhere to a regimen. One man with emphysema was not supposed to smoke or drink. On vacation with friends he lapsed and did both. Upon reflection he was discouraged, thinking he could never fully adhere. Yet in discussions with his physician he was able to identify factors that had led him to abandon his regimen, develop strategies to avoid problems in the future, and return to his regimen. Falling off a regimen, even for an extended period of time, does not mean that one cannot return to it.

Partnership also involves respecting individual choices. For example, there may be cases in which individuals wish to attempt alternate, nontraditional therapies such as diets or imagery. When such therapies offer no recognizable harm and they are complementary to rather than competitive with conventional therapies, they should not be discouraged. Participating in such therapies may provide an ill individual with a renewed sense of control and hope. Respecting individuals' choices and seeking to facilitate them, for example, by accommodating diets in hospitalizations, may enhance coping and encourage general adherence with the medical regimen since it reinforces the full partnership in treatment.

There may also be situations where individuals make a decision not to adhere to treatment or to try a competitive nontraditional therapy. When such cases involve competent adults, caregivers can explore with individuals the reasons for and the risks associated with such decisions. In some cases, an individual's reluctance to accept treatment may involve depression, anxieties, or other feelings that can be addressed, or misinformation that can be corrected. Other times individuals may distrust the medical establishment and feel that it has little to offer; thus they feel that little will be risked in trying something different. Again it is worthwhile to explore these feelings. In other cases, compromises or simplifications of the regimen may resolve concerns.

There may be situations, though, that are not so readily resolved. Here an individual has made, in his or her terms, a rational decision, perhaps a very different one than a caregiver or a family member might make, not to adhere with a part of the regimen, to end treatment, or to seek unconventional therapy. For example, in one case, a sixty-year-old man with leukemia who had already survived two prior (and unrelated to this occurrence) bouts with cancer, decided to forego further chemotherapy for this third encounter with malignancy. He reasoned that the treatment would impair any remaining time he had while promising only limited opportunity for success. Such decisions have to be respected. But caregivers and counselors should encourage individuals to explore reasons for the decision, to discuss its effects on family, and to review other possible options for treatment.

Sometimes people decide not to participate in conventional therapies because they believe "nothing can be done." They need to be convinced that things *can* be done within the context of conventional medicine, perhaps not to cure, but possibly to extend life, to alleviate symptoms, and/or to control pain. Physicians and other caregivers must encourage openness, for only when the individual expresses his or her true feelings and beliefs can they be addressed.

Caregivers can often be threatened, even personally offended, by a person's decision to seek alternate therapies. The most helpful approach for physicians and other caregivers, however, is to discuss in a nondefensive manner the reasons for an individual's decision and to provide the invitation and freedom for that person to return to more conventional treatments should they someday desire.

In summary, adherence should be regarded as a continuum. On one end are those who fully adhere. On the other end are those who do not adhere at all. Most will be between these poles, adhering to varying degrees. Understanding where one is in that continuum, what factors influence the degree of compliance, what risks and benefits are associated with the present state of adherence, and what one can do to maintain and/or enhance adherence with caregivers often helps. This ongoing assessment of adherence also provides continued opportunities to receive education and instruction. Often at the beginning of treatment anxiety levels are high and the information and instruction presented may be overwhelming. Hence, periodic assessments provide a better opportunity to review techniques of treatment, answer questions, and to discuss any difficulties. When individuals have difficulty with adherence, caregivers may wish to explore factors and situations that inhibit adherence. However, caregivers and family members should remember that certain behaviors such as exhortations, "all or nothing" comments (for example, "Will you follow the diet or not?"), or threatening comments (for example, "If you don't follow this regimen you will surely relapse!") are not likely to be effective in improving adherence. Adherence will be improved in a context that emphasizes full partnership, honesty, good communication, clear empathy, and mutual respect.

Preventing and Managing Medical Crises

The chronic phase is often punctuated by a variety of medical crises. If these crises are poorly managed they can adversely affect both physical and mental health. Effective prevention and management of medical crises, on the other hand, can often reaffirm a sense of control and raise morale.

Caregivers can assist individuals in preventing medical crises through careful observation and education. Individuals should discuss with their physician potential danger signs and symptoms that mandate immediate attention. This can become a useful opportunity to assess symptoms, strategies, and possible difficulties that may arise. By paying prompt attention to potential problems, carefully adhering to treatment regimen, and maintaining an effective life-style, an ill individual can prevent many crises.

But not all medical crises can be avoided. It often helps to do some contingency planning with caregivers and family that identifies possible sources of informal support and medical assistance. For example, you may need to know who to contact if the primary physician is not readily available. If you are traveling, you may need the names of local physicians and medical centers should emergencies arise. If you live alone, you may wish to arrange for someone to call every day at a certain time to make sure you're OK.

Developing a flow chart can be a very effective technique for both individuals and their families. Here physicians and other caregivers identify possible medical contingencies and difficulties and outline appropriate responses. In some cases the action may be as mild as "inform the physician at the next visit"; in other cases the action to be taken may be to seek immediate emergency care. One side benefit of such a flow chart is to reassure the ill individual that not every symptom or event constitutes a major crisis. Families can add their own notes: who can be contacted, who can provide needed support (for example, transportation, meals, and the like), who else should be notified. These charts should be kept in a place familiar and available to other family members. Such a chart can forestall a sense of panic that can immobilize people in a chronic phase.

Crisis planning is best done in a noncrisis context, early in the chronic phase. When creating a contingency list, it is important to remind all concerned that these events are contingencies that might *possibly* occur, not sure predictions. Making the list or flow chart should be an interactive process with families fully participating. Many find this kind of planning hopeful, since it emphasizes all the actions that one can take to prevent and control possible crises. But others feel threatened by addressing future crises. If this process begins to seem too threatening, one can merely list and post medical personnel that should be contacted should need arise.

Managing Stress and Examining Coping

Living with disease is quite stressful because the individual is trying to maintain a quality of life with varying degrees of diminished capacity, energy, and resources, as well as pain, psychological distress, and the increased demands of treatment. Often life in the chronic phase is full of small crises, constant problems with which the individual must deal. Managing stress is often a critical problem.

It is helpful to begin to deal with this problem by assessing both current sources and symptoms of stress as well as styles of coping with stress. It often is useful to think about earlier challenges and crises that were resolved successfully. Not only can such a mental review enhance coping by reminding one of past successful coping skills, it can also reduce anxiety by reminding one of the times one has surmounted prior problems. One should consider the ways that current life-style and current state of disease may inhibit or facilitate effective stress management. Proper diet, activity, exercises, diversion, even humor, may be adaptive mechanisms that can help build stress resistance. Counselors may also be able to teach effective techniques for stress reduction such as biofeedback, relaxation, or meditation. The ill individual would do well to identify, alter, and avoid situations that exacerbate stress.

In this period one may have to challenge one's own unrealistic expectations. One cannot do everything that one did prior to the illness. It is important to recognize that energy is going to be expended in fighting the illness even when symptoms are not apparent. If one is coping with time-consuming treatments, disruptive symptoms, or even increased fatigue, maintaining previous activities and involvements is even harder. In these circumstances, surrendering certain activities or delegating responsibilities may help to reduce stress. When these measures are only marginally effective and stress levels remain so high that health or sleep is adversely affected, one's physician may decide to recommend medication.

However, there are alternatives to medication that one may wish to try. One woman unable to sleep well since her diagnosis was reluctant to take sleeping pills both because she had younger children (and feared she wouldn't wake up if they needed her) and because she wanted to minimize any drugs she was taking. She found sleep-relaxation tapes a helpful alternative.

Since stress levels will fluctuate considerably during the chronic phase, stress should be constantly monitored throughout the illness.

Maximizing Social Support and Minimizing Social Isolation

During the chronic phase individuals and their families may experience a deep sense of social isolation. Often individuals and families have the perception that social support is more readily available in times of crisis such as the initial diagnosis.

There are many reasons for this perception. In the context of a clear crisis, need may be more apparent and appropriate ways to respond more clearly defined. If someone is hospitalized, friends have clear norms about what they are expected to do. But when an individual returns home, friends may be unaware of the continued needs of the patient and uncomfortable or unclear about what they should say or do. Other factors too may contribute to a sense of isolation. Separation from work or recreational roles may limit opportunities for interaction. The financial pressures of chronic illness as well as decreased energy levels or other symptoms of disease may also decrease individual and family interactions with others. Fears may further isolate the individual, as friends and family avoid patients, and become worried, often needlessly, about possible contagion.

The ill individual needs to assess who in his network of family and friends can and does provide support. He can begin by listing the names of those persons he believes can be counted on. Often this simple act can give a person a comforting sense of just how extensive his network is. The individual may also wish to explore variables such as geographic distance, other roles, and obligations that might affect the ability of members in the network to provide support. He may wish to examine the different relationships he has with varied members that may affect the level of perceived support. For example, some family members and close friends may have extensive ties, bound by mutual obligations, affections, and past support. With other persons, ties and expectations of support may have to be more limited. Once the network is defined, an individual can assess the ways that he is using his network. Sometimes the problem is that others may not be able to provide the help you need. They may, though, be more comfortable in assisting in other ways.

Reviewing one's network may also mitigate another potential problem. Some individuals, particularly older persons or individuals with younger families or dependent members, may have serious concerns about how others will survive their death. Reviewing one's network can be a useful way to build reassurance that the needs of others will continue to be met even if one should become seriously incapacitated or die.

It is also important to avoid social isolation as much as possible. One may begin by assessing one's degree of involvement prior to the illness as well as the changes that occurred after diagnosis. This can suggest factors that contribute to isolation. Again, these factors can be varied and can include physical incapacitation, stigma, immobility, shrinking social roles, others' discomfort, fears or anxieties, or other psychological factors that inhibit interaction. Once these factors are identified, one can begin to develop strategies to lessen this social isolation and reengage in social life.

Throughout this exploration one needs to remember that there is an important distinction between isolation, which is an objective state, and loneliness which is a subjective feeling. One can be relatively isolated, having few opportunities for interaction, but not feel lonely. Or one can be isolated and lonely. One can have considerable interaction with others but still feel a deep sense of loneliness. This last state often reflects situations where one interacts extensively but still feels that basic needs are unmet. And this too reinforces the connection between issues of isolation and support.

Finally, one may identify sources of formal support to complement and supplement informal networks. These can include social service agencies, disease-related organizations, such as the American Cancer Society, and self-help groups. Self-help groups can be particularly helpful in providing both resources of social support and activities and interactions that ease social isolation.

Normalizing Life in the Face of Disease

The central difficulty in the chronic phase is living with the disease. As the chronic phase begins, one must try to accommodate the demands of daily life to the new reality of that disease. This struggle continues throughout the chronic phase, especially if further deterioration raises new complications.

Roles, relationships, and identity are often the major issues in attempting to maintain a normal life. Throughout the chronic phase the disease can constantly assault a sense of self. Symptoms can be so intrusive that they may impair the ways you look at yourself and how you relate to others. One's sense of sexual identity and sexual relationships may be affected as well. Others can react with embarrassment, awkwardness, or even rejection, not knowing how to relate to the person. Important roles may be compromised by the nature of the disease, its symptoms, and treatment. The ill individual may be unable to function effectively in school, at work, or in other significant roles. Living a life as normal as possible is a key challenge of chronic illness. One of the first things that one can do is to fully explore the ways the disease has affected one's life. Consider the effects of the disease on sense of self, roles, and relationships.

One of the biggest changes may be in one's sexual relationship. Health, body image, self-concept, relationships with others, and sexuality are all closely associated. Changes in one area may affect all the others. For example, declines in health or certain forms of treatment may affect sexual desires or performance. Changes in body images such as scarring, particularly when it occurs in parts of the body associated with sexuality, may have similar effects. Even the attitude of one's partner can be affected by the disease. For example, one woman was reluctant to have sexual relationships with her husband following his heart attack. She believed that the excitement would endanger his health. Her anxiety affected her sexual desire, and ultimately her relationship with her husband.

The key to resolving sexual difficulties lies in honest communication. First, that means establishing honest communication with physicians and other medical caregivers. When I train caregivers I stress the importance of taking a good sexual history of patients and periodically monitoring the effects of the illness on sexual behaviors and relationships. Patients should be encouraged to discuss their sex lives by the caregiver. Often such discussion can clear up any myths or misunderstandings that might be impairing sexual expression. Similarly, self-help groups or counselors can also be helpful in examining the ways that an illness might influence sexuality.

Of course, honest communication is essential between ill individuals and their partners. Each needs to openly share feeling and experiences, what is comfortable and what causes discomfort. Often we are so uncomfortable with our own sexuality that we avoid such conversations. But this open sharing can resolve difficulties. Sometimes patience and compromise are also necessary. One woman, for example, was reluctant to undress in front of her husband following a mastectomy. He constantly reassured her that her operation made no difference to him. He found himself angry and frustrated that she did not accept his assurance, while she felt pressured. In counseling they were able to reach some compromises. She recognized their needs for intimacy and her husband recognized her need for privacy at this point in her life. She undressed privately and in the dark. Recognizing her needs, he no longer felt that his assurances were ignored.

This case also illustrates two additional points. First, sometimes counseling can be very effective in assisting couples as they examine their sexual relationships during the course of illness. Second, couples can sometimes learn through a counseling process that sexual intimacy is multifaceted and doesn't always have to be expressed through sexual intercourse. This can be particularly critical if the illness has affected sexual performance, or, as in a disease such as AIDS, made sexual acts that involve the exchanging of body fluids dangerous. One man once told me that one of the most erotic and intimate experiences he ever experienced was his wife's gentle massaging and kissing at a time when he was too frail for other sexual acts.

Other roles and relationships may change as well. In focusing on the ways that the disease has changed one's life, one can determine factors that inhibit normalcy and develop creative solutions to difficulties. For example, one man who had returned to work while he was struggling with cancer believed that his supervisors were being overprotective, sheltering him from work challenges that he felt would be a welcome diversion. In counseling he explored his own reasoning as well as that of his supervisors. He role-played various ways that he might approach them until he found an approach that he thought would be both personally comfortable and effective. He then was able to resolve his work difficulties. Families and friends may be overprotective, perhaps even overbearing, inhibiting one from reaching one's potential and sometimes even inducing dependency.

In other cases, though one may be reluctant to accept the fact, the continued deterioration of health or the demands of treatment may have made the continuance of a previous life-style difficult if not impossible. Here one may need to realistically explore what roles can be maintained and what roles will have to be modified or even surrendered. In some cases one may discover alternate opportunities that allow one to maintain, perhaps in limited fashion, important roles. In one case, for example, a college professor, already on reduced load, was reluctant to give up his two last classes. His dean, however, was deeply concerned both that he was so debilitated that teaching would be difficult and that he very well might not survive until the end of the semester. As the dean and professor discussed their mutual concerns and needs, they were able to devleop an effective solution: both courses would be team taught with an adjunct (or part-time) instructor selected by that professor.

Not every situation can be so easily resolved. Decisions to leave work can be constrained by financial reasons. One young man who had developed a form of muscular dystrophy in his twenties found that the physical demands of his work increased his sense of weakness and fatigue. Although he was in the early stages of the disease, his physician advised him to take a less-physical job. However, given his lack of education, only construction work paid a wage that allowed him to maintain his financial independence. Leaving this work provided stark alternatives: he would lose his medical insurance, and he would also have to return to a conflicted home that he had left only two years earlier. Even telling his boss about his condition did not seem viable to him since he doubted whether he would be permitted to keep his job were his condition known.

Often self-help groups can be effective resources in assisting one in normalizing life. Support and self-help groups can often provide "tricks of the trade" or strategies that one can use in normalizing life. In addition, they can offer acceptance, moral support, and models of successful adjustment. Often they are reservoirs of creative and effective problem solving. However, everyone has to make a decision as to whether such groups are personally helpful. For some, these groups may reinforce an unpleasant sense of being different.

The key to normalizing life in the face of disease lies in negotiating the conflicts between one's wants, one's needs, and one's abilities. Begin by recognizing what one wants to do, what one needs to do in order to maintain a quality of life, and what one is able to do at this point in the illness. Once these wants, needs, and abilities have been clarified, strive to find creative solutions that allow living as normally as possible with the constraints posed by the disease and treatment.

Dealing with Financial Concerns

The most significant stress within the chronic period is often financial. Life-threatening illness often has adverse financial effects. Medical bills mount, just as income is reduced. Incidental expenses are legion, including transportation to and from hospitals, meals eaten out in the course of visits and treatment, special diet supplements, perhaps increased childcare costs, environmental modifications, and even such things as new clothing perhaps necessitated by significant changes in weight or other physical symptoms of the disease.

Four approaches may assist in helping to cope with financial difficulties:

It often helps just to become aware of the costs of illness. In many cases one may be experiencing financial pressure and may not yet have identified the increased demands that cause it. Often just listing the money spent on incidental expenses in a given time period can be a revelation. Once these costs are determined, one can develop a budget. In some cases this may be the first time one has even had a need to budget.

One may want to identify possible resources within one's circle of family and friends as well as community resources. Transportation costs might be reduced if one used friends or community resources for rides. The local cancer society may, for example, provide transportation at little or no cost. If eating out costs too much, one can pack a lunch. Understanding what the illness actually costs can help one plan alternate strategies for reducing cost.

One may also need to identify and explore one's resistance and reluctance to utilize social services or support. Americans like to think of themselves as self-sustaining and independent. These beliefs might become even stronger during life-threatening illness. With everything else in disarray and while coping with physical dependency, it can be difficult to recognize another form of dependency. Yet it is precisely at this time that one may need help most. One always has to review when independence is functional and when it is not functional. Again, sometimes counselors can help explore this and even serve as advocates in arranging supportive services.

Finally, sometimes the services of financial planners can be helpful in assisting one in making decisions on how and when to tap into financial resources. Sometimes one may need their help to learn how to set up journals to document medical and related expenses for tax purposes.

Again, these decisions are not purely financial. Selling stocks or annuities may also involve letting go of future dreams. Estate planning can reaffirm one's own mortality and occasionally reopen old issues. One client, for example, was reluctant to sign a will since he had hoped to include a bequest to a sister. But he was unwilling to make such a bequest since they were still unreconciled. Yet not to include her in the will suggested an unwelcome finalization of their present alienation. In summary, then, financial and estate planning, necessitated by the current illness, can raise psychological and relational issues that one may need to address. Understanding that discomfort, and exploring it with family or counselors, is part of this process.

One of the more difficult financial problems may involve health insurance coverage. Even with insurance, the costs of a major illness can be staggering. Because many insurance companies are trying to control these costs, they may challenge certain costs incurred by individuals. For example, many insurance companies may refuse to pay for treatments they regard as experimental.

Insurance hassles can be highly upsetting. They can become one more stressful thing to deal with, generating strange feelings of anxiety, anger, even betrayal. Yet try to remain calm. Individuals have rights in dealing with medical insurance under the Employment Retirement Insurance Security Act (ERISA). One's insurance agent or benefits coordinator will have information about ERISA. Discuss what documentation is needed with the benefits coordinator, your insurance agent, or the insurance company's claims representative. As a last alternative, seek legal advice.

Preserving Self-Concept

Sometimes in the chronic phase individuals will begin to internalize a self-definition that includes the disease and deterioration experienced. To many people the central aspect of their self-concept is now that they are "a person with a disease," different and stigmatized by that fact. I remember one twelve-year-old boy who had leukemia. At the time he was in remission and as active as any young adolescent. Nothing in his appearance indicated the disease, but its impact was seared into his psyche. He frequently began conversations with the phrase "When I was normal . . . ," thereby revealing the degree to which the presence of disease was now a central part of how he viewed himself.

The more one continues prior activities, the easier it is to preserve one's self-concept. Some individuals also find it helpful to use varied techniques to preserve their physical self-concept. For example, if one loses hair in chemotherapy, wearing a wig may help. Finally, families and caregivers can have a significant role in preserving an individual's sense of self. For the more caregivers and family members treat a person as normal, the easier it is for that person to maintain a sound sense of self.

Redefining Relationships with Others throughout the Course of the Disease

During the chronic phase the effects of the disease may also impinge on the ill person's interactions with others. Life-threatening illness has the potential to severely affect social relationships. Others who know the diagnosis may have difficulty interacting with someone who is both seriously ill but still appears healthy and vigorous. Preston (1979) discusses what he calls the "Gregor effect." He draws from Kafka's famous story "Metamorphosis," in which the protagonist, Gregor, wakes up one morning to find himself transformed into a giant cockroach. But it is his family's subsequent treatment of him as an insect that really modifies his own self-perception. Their behavior reinforces this new reality. Treated differently he becomes different. The "Gregor effect" implies that the diagnosis of disease becomes a stigma, a mark that impinges on all other social roles and affects all other relationships and interactions. In her book *The Private Worlds of Dying Children*, Myra Bluebond-Langner (1978, p. 172) notes this change: "Until the diagnosis was made (about the second or third day after admission), the children were, in their own eyes and in the eyes of their parents, not different from other children. . . . Once the diagnosis was made, however, everything changed. People, especially the family, started to treat the children differently, who then noticed the change." In short, the presence of life-threatening illness can change relationships with others. The new status, the illness role produced by the diagosis, adds uncertainty to every relationship and every other role. These changes can continue throughout the course of the illness.

The key issue here is to recognize that every significant change in one's life has a ripple effect that influences every other part of life, including every relationship. Life-threatening illness is a significant change, one that generates many ripples.

It is important to understand the ways in which the illness has affected other relationships. Perhaps others are uncomfortable. Not knowing what is expected of them, or how to act, they may either avoid one who is ill or act differently. Here, honest communication sometimes can help. In other cases, people may not be able to handle the illness. In some cases, changed situations, such as leaving a work role, can change relationships. Without the common bond, the relationship may not generate the interest or time to sustain itself. A philosophical attitude sometimes can help. One man undergoing treatment for cancer expressed it well. "There are," he said, "some friends who are there for me when I'm sick. Others who are there for me when I'm better. I've learned to treasure both."

Ventilating Feelings and Fears

At every phase of illness one has to cope with many feelings and fears. These feelings and fears may be quite varied, and include many of the responses I noted in Chapter 1. One should be aware that the nature and the intensity of these feelings may vary with the course and trajectory of the illness.

Often these feelings will intensify at crisis points within the illness or in periods characterized by continued deterioration. At such times fears and feelings associated with disability, dependency, and dying may loom large, perhaps even becoming overwhelming. In such periods all assumptions, rationalizations, and other defenses may be challenged. For example, one may reassure oneself that if one adheres to the treatment, or continues certain activities such as prayer or meditation, or changes behaviors, the illness will be arrested. This defense may allow one to effectively defend against the disease for a while and resume a normal life. But physical deterioration or a medical crisis can overwhelm such a defense, generating strong affect and anxieties.

Different types of treatments can be associated with changes in affect or anxiety. In some cases treatment may ease primary or secondary emotional side effects. For example, depression may be a side effect of some medications, and others can cause include fatigue and irritability, which can translate into such feelings as depression or anger. Hospitalization too, even if routine, can reinforce fears of dependency and death. One may exhibit a great deal of ambivalence about treatment even when the treatment seems relatively unobtrusive, routine, and successful. One may worry about the psychological and financial costs of one's illness to one's families.

Even at times in the illness when one is in remission, one may still experience many emotions and anxieties. One may be unrealistically optimistic, anxious, irritable, highly depressed, or have any variety of possible responses. The very fact that things are going well may make one anxious, causing one to look for bad news or an expected blow. The point is that one should not assume in these relatively tranquil periods that one will be free of emotional stress. These reactions and responses are normal during any phase of the illness. In fact, in seemingly tranquil periods one may have more time to reflect upon feelings and fears. During this time too one may have less emotional support from others who may be constantly encouraging one not to think negatively, thereby denying one's honest and natural emotional responses.

Since the course of disease is likely to change, one needs to adjust to the constant changes posed by the disease. Whenever one experiences these changes, it is important to discuss one's feelings and fears, particularly the meanings that one gives to such changes. Perhaps the change is viewed as only a temporary setback. Or perhaps the change is perceived as an ominous omen, foreshadowing continued decline and eventual death, dashing any hope of recovery or even relative stability. These meanings may not be the same meanings that caregivers place upon the change. But in any case, it may help to review with caregivers the changes and their meanings, assess the validity of one's concerns and fears, consider the effects these changes will have upon one's life, and determine strategies for dealing with these changes. In addition, with every significant change in illness, one may need to review the viability of any previous decisions, for example, whether or not to work, and to reconsider contingency plans.

However, effects may not be as radical as one initially fears. Discussing and exploring the significance of each change during illness leads to greater understanding on the part of the patient, family, and caregivers. This understanding may alleviate anxiety, suggest more effective strategies for coping, and facilitate any decisions that one needs to make.

Thus, throughout the chronic phase, caregivers should allow and encourage their patients to ventilate and explore their emotions in a nonjudgmental and accepting atmosphere. And because feelings and fears may vary considerably, depending on the nature and course of the disease, others should follow the ill individual's lead. It is not unusual that individuals ride an emotional roller coaster, shifting back and forth between times when they feel positive and upbeat, and other times when they feel depressed, angry, or lonely.

In some cases just ventilating these emotions may allow you a sense of resolution and comfort. Often it is very helpful to have a confidant who has the ability to simply listen. Many times family members can be too threatened by your illness to assume that role. It can be hard for them to listen to your pain quietly. They may have a need to constantly reassure both you and themselves that everything will be all right. A confidant's value lies in the fact that you can unburden yourself and explore your deepest fears and strongest feelings. Find a person who is both trustworthy and accepting, who listens to feelings rather than attempting to talk you out of those feelings. Counselors also fulfill that role, but few have the confidant's inclination to listen at 2:00 A.M. in the morning. In summary, special friends, confidants, counselors, and caregivers can be valued resources as one works through all the complex reactions that may emerge in this chronic period.

In other cases listening may not be enough. Individuals may need to develop ways to resolve their emotional conflicts or to develop strategies for handling their anxieties and feelings more effectively. In one case a thirty-year-old Hispanic male with testicular cancer was deeply troubled and consumed by guilt, attributing the disease to sexual sins. Encouraged to explore ways of resolving that intense guilt, he reached back to his past religious traditions, engaging in the sacrament of Confession with a sympathetic priest. Following his penance and absolution, he felt emotionally healed. In another case a fifty-year-old female battling cancer, was able to recognize her anger and its effects on her family, and to develop alternative strategies—in her case, pounding on dough—to diffuse her feelings.

Finding Meaning in Suffering, Chronicity, Uncertainty, or Decline

The chronic phase has a number of possible resolutions. In some cases treatment, although it may have been long and painful, can produce a total cure. Some ill individuals may experience a partial recovery. In other cases the condition can stabilize, leading the individual to experience an extended period of chronic illness and ongoing uncertainty. And finally, some will experience continued decline.

Each of these circumstances raises continued issues that individual and families need to explore. Even in recovery, discussed in the next chapter, there may be deep anxiety about reoccurrences of the disease. For example, individuals may be ambivalent about terminating relationships with specialists who may have followed their cases for as long as a decade. Many factors may be operating here—a strong, close bond, perhaps a magical sense of protection. Caregivers may not always recognize the strong bond that individuals and their families may feel for them and the ambivalence they feel about leaving. Thus caregivers expecting and exuding delight in the cure may unwillingly contribute to a sense of abandonment. Individuals may wish to examine their life-style, maximizing healthful practices that minimize chances of reoccurrence or new disease. They may need to review their former aspirations as a prelude to rebuilding their life. And they may have a need to interpret and integrate the illness in their lives to consider what the experience has meant for them.

With continued chronicity and uncertainty, individuals may have to constantly rework issues and tasks raised within the chronic phase. They may need assistance in understanding the peculiar stresses of long-term uncertainty and the implications of that uncertainty for their behaviors and relationships. Such uncertainty may impair any ability to plan. Hypersensitivity and distrust may be generated by long periods of uncertainty. Some may believe information is being withheld and scrutinize every remark of both family and caregiving staff searching for clues. They may have a sense that the illness is taking too much time, and become angry, depressed, or resigned.

Whatever the experience of illness, the ill person has a need to try to understand and interpret that experience. "Why am I suffering?" "Why did this happen to me?" "Why did it happen now?" These questions are attempts to struggle with the meaning of the disease, or even more fundamentally with issues of purpose and meaning in life or death. Each individual will need to struggle with these questions on his or her own, either answering the questions in a way that is personally meaningful or deciding that these questions are ultimately unanswerable. Sometimes discussing these issues with a counselor or a member of the clergy, or reading a book such as Kushner's (1981) *When Bad Things Happen to Good People* can provide opportunities for reflection and insight.

In summary, the chronic phase is a long, uncertain, and difficult period for both individuals and their families. But it is also a time of opportunity—opportunity to fight to get well, opportunity to make the best of the time that one has, opportunity to live and experience life in its fullest sense even when fighting off disease and possible death.

6

Coping with Recovery

At any phase in life-threatening illness a partial or full recovery may occur. Perhaps the original diagnosis was wrong or too pessimistic. In other cases initial treatment may be successful in effecting a cure, perhaps immediately following the diagnosis or after a chronic phase. Even in the terminal phase a recovery may be experienced. Recoveries may be partial or complete. In some cases one may retain no apparent ill effects from the disease. In other cases, however, one may experience diminished abilities, carry physical scars, or bear psychological injuries.

"Recovery" and "cure" are perhaps the most welcome words in life-threatening illness. I remember the great sense of celebration when we learned my father would fully recover. Happily, these words are used more and more often. However, it is important to recognize that while these words are used more often, recovery does not mean that one simply returns to the life led before. Any encounter with a crisis changes us. We are no longer the people we once were. Even a recovery leaves certain issues that have to be explored and tasks that need to be completed as one attempts to move one with one's life.

Dealing with the Physical, Psychological, Social, Financial, and Spiritual Residues of Illness

There are often a series of aftereffects to life-threatening illness and treatment. There may be physical scars or permanent disabilities. One may need to develop responses to these physical effects. One may also have to grieve secondary losses that result from these physical changes. One young woman whose leg was amputated, for example, grieved the loss of her athletic career. This activity had been both an important part of her self-identity and the center of her social life and friendships. Others often invalidated these expressions of grief, reminding her that a leg was a small price to pay for recovery. While this sentiment may be true, it did not make her loss any less real. Once the crisis of the illness was over, she was left to consider that cost. Only now, once the threat was over, could she realize what she had lost and grieve about the way her life had changed. She recognized that her sense of self-identity was changed by her bout with life-threatening illness.

There may be other emotional and social scars as well. One may continue to experience a range of emotional responses, often including anger and guilt. One may be angry that one had suffered, guilty about life-style factors that one believes contributed to the illness, even guilty over recovery.

There may be social disruptions as well. One may feel disappointed by the responses of family and friends. In some cases spouses or lovers who were supportive during the crisis may feel free to leave now. Friends too may feel uncomfortable with the recovered person, perhaps even fearing disease. Or recovered individuals may find their friends' concerns trivial or unimportant. After a bout with cancer or another life-threatening illness, it can be hard to be sympathetic when friends or families experience seemingly minor problems. One client shared with me her friend's exasperation. She would always try to comfort her friend with the comment, "Well, at least it's not life-threatening." After a particularly difficult day, her friend rebuked her, saying, "Do I have to have cancer to get sympathy and support?" The incident reminded my client both of the perspective she had gained from her illness and her need to be aware of others' needs.

Some may find it difficult to establish new intimate relationships, perhaps because they fear the future. Others may be reluctant to become involved with someone they fear may become ill.

Employment and careers can also be changed by the illness. One may have lost or left a job during the illness. Coworkers may be fearful. One may encounter discrimination because of medical history that affects the ability to obtain a position, change jobs, or advance. Some people may experience demotions or dismissals.

There may be financial effects. Obtaining life insurance or medical insurance may be difficult. One may have exhausted savings and piled up considerable debts.

There often are spiritual residues to life-threatening illness. One's sense of security may be threatened. The way one looks at life may change. One's faith and beliefs may be altered. Some may find a deeper sense of spirituality, while others find their religious perspectives challenged.

These effects can sometimes be long lasting. A colleague of mine and his wife decided not to have children. He had had extensive chemotherapy and radiation treatments during a struggle with cancer during adolescence, and so he and his wife feared possible birth defects. While this fear may or may not have been realistic, it does illustrate how one's encounter with life-threatening illness may affect decisions and choices even decades later.

Counseling can be very helpful during the recovery phase, providing there is an opportunity for individuals to explore these remaining issues. Often it is helpful just to have concerns recognized and validated. Many times individuals who have recovered from life-threatening illness are made to feel ungrateful if they complain. After all, they are told, they are lucky to be alive. This may be true, and most individuals recognize this truth, but it still does not change the fact that illness and recovery extracted a fearful price. I have found that just asking clients about the effects of an illness—all the effects, physical, psychological, social, spiritual, and financial—reassures them that it is acceptable, even in recovery, to recognize the high and continued cost of illness.

Once these concerns are recognized and explored, one can develop ways to deal with them. Perhaps one can discuss concerns with family, friends, clergy, or coworkers. In some cases there may be administrative or legal remedies to particular problems such as job or insurance discrimination. It is important that each individual make decisions about the ways to handle these aftereffects of illness that are comfortable for him or her. Not every solution will be the same for everyone. For example, some individuals will find prosthesis or reconstructive surgery important to their sense of normalcy and their own self-image, while others may find reconstruction or prosthetic devices unnecessary.

Self-help groups such as Cancervive for persons who have recovered from life-threatening illness can also be helpful. These support groups can help individuals realize they are not alone in coping with their concerns. The stories and accounts of other members may provide ongoing inspiration as well as successful strategies for dealing with the problems that persist in recovery.

Coping with Ongoing Fears and Anxieties, Including Fear of Reoccurrence

It is very normal and natural following an experience with life-threatening illness for an individual to continue to have a strong sense of anxiety, depression, or other similar reactions. There are a number of reasons for this. An experience with life-threatening illness reminds one of the fragility of life. It heightens a sense of vulnerability. It reminds one how quickly illness or death can threaten.

Second, the individual may experience continued anxiety about recovery and activity. What can one do? How much should one attempt? What is really pushing the limit? Is this recovery progressing at an expected and/or acceptable pace? These questions can continue for a considerable period of time after a recovery. Sociologist Rodney Coe (1970) once compared recovery to adolescence, describing it as a continuous, often anxiety-ridden, test of reemerging strength against ongoing, increasing life demands.

Finally, there may also be high anxiety about the reoccurrence of illness. Individuals may be highly sensitive toward symptoms that are associated with the return of illness. For example, a woman who had recovered from cancer particularly feared stomach pains since she believed such pain was a likely sign of metastasis. Many persons who have recovered from life-threatening illness suffer anxiety whenever they have a routine doctor's appointment. One woman who had recovered from cancer told me that she had a panic attack every year before her annual checkup with the oncologist. Recovered heart patients may be very anxious about chest pains, arm pains, fatigue, shortness of breath, or other related symptoms; recovered stroke victims may be highly agitated by symptoms associated with stroke such as numbness, headaches, or blurred vision.

There are a number of ways to deal with these fears. It is important to discuss these anxieties with others. Do not hold them inside. Sometimes it is easy to fall into superstitious beliefs when dealing with fears: we may feel that if we express them, they may occur. Talking fears over with others will allow one to evaluate one's fears. It is especially helpful to express these concerns to a physician. Often physicians can provide helpful information about the pace of recovery or the real risks of reoccurrence. They can also help one to assess changes in life-style or preventive health behaviors that might minimize chances of reoccurrence or new disease. These changes may also give one a renewed sense of control that lessens feelings of vulnerability.

Many individuals may also find imagery and meditation useful. Imaging continued health and recovery, taking time to relax and meditate, pursuing diversion and exercise are all ways to reduce anxiety, manage stress, and reaffirm personal well-being.

Self-help groups may also be valuable. They can allow opportunities to discuss and to explore concerns in a trusting and accepting atmosphere. Again, other survivors can provide reassuring role models.

Examining Life and Life-Style Issues and Reconstructing One's Life

One of the natural desires in recovery is to turn the clock back, to go back to the way things were prior to the illness. While this is a natural and normal wish, it is unlikely to be achieved. Often too much has occurred during the illness, changing both recovered individuals and their families, to simply resume earlier patterns of life. One needs to recognize that while one cannot go back to the way things were, one can establish a new life-style with a different and new sense of normalcy.

The illness may have changed relationships with family or friends. Each person affected by the illness has changed, and perhaps grown as well. For example, children may have learned to be more independent during the course of a mother or father's illness. Often family roles also may have changed. In one case a young wife took on increased responsibilities for the family's business when her husband became ill. Following his recovery, she had no desire to relinquish her interest in that business.

Sometimes a return to the past may not even be desirable. Perhaps poor health or life-style practices contributed to the illness. For example, in one case a forty-one-year-old man had to realize that a return to his previous stress-ridden job and unhealthy life-style would likely re-create, in short order, the conditions that led to his heart attack. Like many persons recovering from illness, he needed to identify and change negative health practices.

Finally, illness sometimes changes one's personal priorities. Things that seemed important in the past may no longer seem so essential now. Many times people will grow through the illness, reestablishing personal priorities. For some an encounter with life-threatening illness can be a positive turning point in life. Joe, a middle-aged man who recovered from cancer, now spends considerably more time with his wife and family. The illness experience reminded him just how important family was to him.

In recovery, it is important to reflect upon and review the illness experience. What has the illness taught? What insights have been gained? Reflection can often help integrate the experience of illness into one's own sense of personal biography. In my counseling with persons who have recovered, I often use three questions that I have adapted from a very special colleague, Dr. Catherine Sanders, who used them in her grief counseling. The questions that I ask clients to reflect upon are:

What do I need to leave behind as I begin this new phase of life?
   This question allows one opportunities to consider the negative residuals of the illness experience. Perhaps there is a sense of vulnerability or anger that one recognizes would impair the sense of restoration and complicate recovery.

What do I want to keep from the illness experience? Not all aspects of the illness experience were likely to have been negative. One may have discovered renewed appreciation of life or family or friends. One may have developed new insights about oneself. One may have identified or improved significant strengths. One may have found renewed faith.

What do I want to add? The illness or its aftermath may have identified certain areas that need to be addressed. In some cases these may result from reordered priorities resulting from the experience. In other cases individuals may no longer have the opportunity to resume old roles, perhaps because of continued physical disabilities or other reasons. Individuals then need to address what new skills, values, or attitudes they may need to adapt to this new world.

One thing is critically important. Avoid rash or overly quick decisions. It is critical to allow time to become aware of the person one has become as a result of the illness, and to adjust to the new realities that exist. One may regret radical changes that are made in the emotional aftermath of recovery. In one case, a fifty-year-old man recovering from cancer wanted to leave his business, return to school, and obtain an education degree. His counselor intervened to help him think more deeply about this change and how it would radically affect his family's financial stability and life-style. Together they also reviewed motivations for the career change, found a program where he could take courses and maintain his job, and thereby plan a much smoother, and almost equally fast, career change.

Redefining Relationships with Caregivers

Throughout the course of the illness one may have forged very close relationships with caregivers. Once one recovers it may be difficult to redefine these relationships or to say goodbye. One may be anxious and resentful that caregivers' attentions begin to focus elsewhere. One may feel a sense of abandonment, perhaps exacerbated by the caregivers' delight in the recovery and kidding comments that there is no longer reason to see one another. Maintenance of the relationship can even have a magical quality to some individuals, who believe that it will ward off reoccurrence.

Families, recovered individuals, and caregivers should avoid abrupt goodbyes. All may need to discuss their feelings about the relationships and ambivalence about termination. Each may wish to validate one another, focusing on what they have learned from the illness struggle. Each may need to redefine the relationship.

Sometimes individuals and families may have a need to acknowledge caregivers by giving appropriate gifts of thanks. This often enables individuals to reciprocate, at least symbolically, the help they have received. While this is understandable and appropriate, it may make some caregivers uncomfortable. In other cases individuals may be hurt or offended if caregivers need to redirect inappropriate gifts. One recovered furrier, for example, wanted to give a favorite nurse a fur coat. She found the gift excessive but was able to suggest giving the coat in her honor to a hospital auction.

Not all situations end so graciously, nor are all feelings so positive. In some cases individuals may have unresolved feelings including anger at staff. Here it may be important to take action that brings a sense of closure. Individuals may wish to discuss their concerns with counselors, caregivers, or administrators. In one case a family was very upset at the emergency room of a local hospital that had misdiagnosed their mother's heart attack. The emergency room had sent her home with a diagnosis of indigestion. Her personal physician insisted, upon hearing the report that same morning, that she meet him at a larger university hospital. His action probably saved her life. Her family decided to deal with their anger by meeting with the local hospital's administrator. When cases do not involve gross unprofessionalism or malpractice, individuals may need to find other ways to bring closure such as perhaps writing a letter that may never be sent, or adding an entry to a journal about their experiences and feelings.

In summary, recovery raises significant issues for individuals and families. Even in recovery there are tasks that must be worked through so that individuals can recover, not only physically, but psychologically, socially, and spiritually as well, and go on to resume changed, but hopefully enhanced, lives.

Facing the Crisis of Death

At a conference I once attended as a student, a speaker described the terminal phase as the time when there is "nothing more to do." Even then, I thought that was a very unfortunate way to view the terminal phase of illness. While there may be little to do to affect a cure or even to prolong life significantly, there is still much that can be done to keep the individual physically comfortable and to provide psychological, social, and spiritual support. Even in this terminal phase, individuals can still live their remaining days with both quality and meaning. For some individuals and their families, the terminal phase can be a significant time, one that allows ill individuals to die with dignity and a sense of completion, one that offers families opportunities to say their good-byes in ways that will ease their deep sense of loss and grief.

This book seeks to address three audiences: ill individuals, their families, and other caregivers. This multiple design is especially appropriate for the topic addressed in this chapter. More than any other time in the illness, the terminal phase is a time when all three groups are intimately connected. When all three groups communicate their needs, and understand their experiences and reactions, they can provide each other with the support that can mean so much during the terminal phase.

I will begin by describing the transition into the terminal phase. I will then review the needs of ill persons and others during this period. I will go on to discuss some difficult decisions that are encountered in the terminal period, such as whether to seek hospice care or when to terminate care-oriented treatment. Even the terminal period has its special tasks. These tasks relate to the challenges presented in this period to the dying person, his or her family, and caregivers.

Understanding the Transition

The terminal phase begins when the medical goal changes from curing a person or maintaining that person in remission to providing palliative or comfort-oriented care. Now the chance of recovery or remission is remote. Death is not only possible, it seems predictable, even imminent.

Usually the terminal phase is first recognized and defined by medical staff. Based on the conditions, symptoms, tests, and responses to treatment, physicians modify their definition of patients from "sick" to "dying." This changed prognosis is usually communicated to other medical staff and even to families and patients through direct means such as physician comments and sometimes through indirect means such as changes in treatment, subtle comments, or even evasions. One man, for example, told me that he first recognized his declining state when his physician ceased making his usual optimistic comments.

Often dying persons do not need a physician's confirmation of their state. Aware of the changes they are undergoing, they sense their impending death. Individuals may have a fair degree of medical knowledge and recognize internal and external cues to their true state.

While individuals, families, and medical staff often share the perception of the transition from ill to dying, this is not always the case. Sometimes the person or the family may be reluctant to admit that the individual is now dying. Other times individuals or their families may perceive that death is near even when medical staff feel that the patient is not dying or when medical staff recognize their patient is dying but still continue, perhaps inappropriately, to treat medically the person as if a cure or significant remission were expected.

In the beginning of this transition to the terminal phase the physical decline of the person may not be perceptible or it may be seen as just another stage in a long continuous decline. The person seems to be slowly fading away. As the physical decline continues, though, it is likely to accelerate and become more noticeable. When family and friends recognize accelerated decline, they focus increased attention on the dying person.

In the final period of the terminal phase individuals may slip in and out of consciousness. By now staff, the family, and often the individual himself or herself recognize that death is near, that the last weeks and days are at hand. This is the period for leave-takings. Family, friends, and staff share their final farewells with the person, sometimes even when the patient is comatose. If the person is conscious, he or she may wish to tie up loose ends. In some religious systems there may be a desire for final rituals such as Last Rites, receiving the Eucharist, or being blessed. Many times dying persons will be granted license to engage in activities formerly forbidden, such as enjoying extra or longer visits, drinking liquor, or smoking cigarettes.

The last moments of the terminal phase have been called the "deathwatch." If staff suspects death is near, family members are notified so that the person does not die alone. Sometimes, though, such predictions are hard to make so that a deathwatch can last much longer than staff anticipated, or the individual may rally and stabilize for a while, leading to a subsequent deathwatch or even a succession of such deathwatches. The terminal phase ends with the pronouncement of death. But this end is simply the beginning of the end of the first phase of the family's grief.

The Dying Individual: Responses and Needs

Awareness of Dying

One of the most valuable exercises I ever experienced was conducted by a colleague, Edie Stark, at a professional conference. Edie asked this assembly of death educators and counselors, "What do dying persons need?" Soon the blackboard was filled with responses: "Understanding," "Honesty," "Good Care," "Touch," "Respect," "Listening," "Contact," "Love," "Relief from Pain," "Diversion," "Humor," and a host of other terms were quickly listed. "Now," Edie continued, "What does a living person need?" Edie had made her point: a list addressed to a living person's needs would be the same. Basic human needs do not change simply because the status or definition of a person changes. As long as we live, certain basic human needs remain the same.

Some human needs, though, are sorely challenged in the terminal phase, often by a misguided sense of protectiveness. One key need that is too often forgotten in this period is the need for honest communication.

In recent years there has been a greater awareness of how individuals understand their own death. Some early studies in this area asked the question, "Do people recognize impending death?" Glaser and Strauss (1965) presented four different conditions of a person's awareness:

1. Closed Awareness—Here the person is unaware of impending death though others could know
2. Suspicion Awareness—The individual suspects that he or she is dying, and often acts to test that suspicion
3. Mutual Pretense—The person and others recognize a dying state but both maintain a pretense that this is not the case
4. Open Awareness—The individual and others recognize and acknowledge to each other that the patient is dying

The researchers found that the last two conditions were likely to be reached even when families and doctors did not share truthful information with the patient, as was often the case at that time. The ill persons themselves still had access to internal clues, and could monitor their own condition. They recognized that they were progressively getting sicker and weaker. They also interpreted external clues: the fact that relatives who lived far away were suddenly dropping in for visits, for example, or that family would respond uncharacteristically to innocent comments. One client told me that his first inkling of impending death occurred when he commented that next spring he wanted to plant an herb garden. His wife grasped his hand tightly, and with tears glistening in her eyes, she cried out "Of course you will." "She never," he wryly commented, "showed much emotion about my gardening." Moreover, ill individuals may have a high degree of sophistication about illness gleaned from interaction with other patients during the course of the illness, their own reading, and TV. Even children, Bluebond-Langner (1978) noted, change their self-concept from one of "very ill, not likely to get better," to "dying" in the final phase of illness.

Discussing Death

The question of whether individuals know and recognize their state is now often moot as a result of changes in medical practice. Most of the early research in this area took place at a time when standard practice was to "protect" the person from the information of impending death. Research (Glaser and Strauss, 1965; Sudnow, 1961; Doka, 1982a) has indicated the impossibility of this task as well as the negative effects of such policies. Often the practice of protection served to further isolate the dying person. For example, I once studied nurses' interactions with dying people in a hospital that discouraged discussions of death. I found nurses often avoided uncomfortable conversations by avoiding dying persons.

In other cases inhibitions on discussions of death impaired the person's ability to finish personal business. When my aunt was dying of cancer, she became insistent about seeing me. I was somewhat surprised by the request because our relationship was cordial but not close. When I arrived at the hospital it was clear that my aunt wanted to see me alone. As my uncle left he whispered that my aunt didn't know she was dying. As soon as he left she turned to me and said, "You know I'm dying." I took her hand and didn't say anything. My silent assent prompted her to make a request. She had become ill right after a move into a new community and she never had the opportunity to formally join a church. She had been active in church all her life and it was important that she die a church member. But whenever she mentioned her desire to her husband, he told her she could join a church once she got well. Her request to see me was a last-ditch effort to break the bonds of pretense.

Due to an increasing recognition of the negative effects of silence, an awareness that dying people need and want to talk about their condition, and a sensitivity to the rights of individuals to know about their condition and participate in their care, there has been a significant change in medical practice. Most physicians are much more open in their communication with dying individuals and their families. Even if physicians do not volunteer or initiate discussions of prognosis, they will respond honestly to patient questions.

Individuals are likely to be aware of their own impending death.

This knowledge, however, may be too horrifying to be constantly confronted. Weisman (1972) suggests that dying persons have a "middle knowledge" of their own death. By that, he means that dying persons sometimes seem to drift in and out of the awareness of death, at times acknowledging its imminence, at other times denying it. The question for Weisman, then, is not, "Does the person know he or she is dying?," but rather, "When, where, to whom, and under what circumstances does a person share knowledge of impending death?"

Dying individuals themselves should be allowed to set the tone for conversation. By their own comments, individuals will indicate what they want to talk about and when it is comfortable to do so. My advice to families and caregivers has always been to do a lot of listening. The goal is to allow for open communication.

Open communication means many things. First, it allows "give and take." Two things can inhibit that process. One is when others take a protective attitude, being reluctant to truly communicate, limiting opportunities for interaction, even employing evasion and deception. Communication, though, can also be inhibited when others overwhelm the patient, answering questions with so much information that the patient cannot digest or even hear all that is said.

In communicating with dying persons there are some key guidelines that should be recognized:

1. *Let the individual set the tone.* Often an individual's questions and comments will indicate what he or she wants to discuss. Because of "middle knowledge," it is important to recognize that these needs may change with different visits, and even with different stages in a single conversation. It is not unusual to have a meaningful conversation about an individual's fears and anxieties about dying one day only to return the next day and discuss a cruise a patient wishes to take when recovered.

Some individuals will chose never to talk about death. One man, recognizing that he had cancer, went over his affairs with family. But from that initial point he made it clear that he wanted to avoid conversations about death. Such defenses as denial or avoidance have to be respected unless they endanger the person or others.

2. *Listen and reflect.* A chaplain told me that one of the most significant encounters she ever had had with a dying person was when

she simply sat and stroked the dying woman's hand while that woman shared her feelings and fears. Many times we find the simple act of listening difficult. We so want to say something, anything, to contribute to the conversation, break the silence, solve the problem, or bring some comfort. Yet often a receptive silence, perhaps combined with some supportive touch, can be far more effective.

Similarly, when we do respond it is often helpful to respond in ways that allow the individual to reflect. Responding to a question such as "Am I going to die?" with another question such as "Are you scared?" conveys the message that one is willing to discuss any concerns, while still allowing the individual the freedom to choose what to talk about. Such a response also permits both the dying person and the other person engaged in conversation an opportunity to really understand what is being asked. Sometimes patients do not really want their questions answered.

3. *Communicate one's own needs.* Not everyone who visits a dying person feels comfortable about discussing death and related topics. If that is your case, it is usually better to communicate such feeling directly to the individual rather than trying to avoid the patient or somehow evade an unsettling topic. Some time ago a friend came to me because she felt she had failed her dying brother. He wanted to talk about his impending death, but she could not bring herself to do it. Finally she said, "Johnny, I want to be here with you and for you, but I can't take these conversations." So instead of talking about death, they talked about the things she could do for him while he was alive. I reassured her that she had not failed her brother at all. She was caring, honest, and there when he needed her.

4. *Remember one's own role.* In court cases hearsay and speculation are not allowed. The same should hold true for communication. Questions best answered by physicians should be directed to them. Encourage direct communication. Sometimes this may mean being an advocate, informing medical personnel of a patient's needs or helping individuals find ways to address their concerns.

5. *Communication is nonverbal as well as verbal.* We can communicate much by our expression and by other nonverbal behavior. Clear discomfort, avoiding patients, limiting opportunities for privacy—all communicate much louder than words a reluctance to hear someone's concerns.

6. *Always allow hope*. In one's responses to dying persons, take care not to extinguish hope. Nothing you say should extinguish the hope that someone holds, however unrealistic it may be. One counseling intern felt that she had violated honest communication because she had responded to a clearly dying person's comment that "I hope I can recover" with the statement, "I hope so too." She had not failed: she had allowed the person to set the tone, and she had responded in a reflective way, with an answer that was sensitive to the patient's own needs at that moment. Moreover, she was kind. One wise instructor once told me "hope should not expire before the patient."

Preserving Autonomy

Related to this need for honest communication is the need to preserve autonomy. Autonomy is often threatened in the terminal phase. Family and staff may make decisions, protectively and somewhat paternalistically, *for* the dying individual instead of *with* that person. Trying to limit stress, families may limit information, filtering out things they believe will upset or trouble the person. This can contribute to the person's isolation and sense of being different. It may further cut the individual off from significant roles. Deprived of information about their children's problems, for example, they may cease feeling like fathers or mothers. Failure to preserve autonomy may further dependency. The point I wish to make is that if dying individuals are prevented from deciding issues for themselves, this denial accentuates the fact that they are dying, robbing them of a sense of dignity.

Preserving and enhancing the basic human need for autonomy reinforces the fact that the person is still living. Open and honest communication provides a context for supportive relationships; allowing the individual to meet the challenges posed in the terminal phase enables him or her to maintain a degree of independence and a strong sense of self.

Spiritual and Existential Needs

Certain needs are accentuated in the terminal phase. Chief among these are spiritual needs.

Often the very fact of death focuses one inward, as one engages in a reflective struggle to meet one's own spiritual needs. These may include three issues. The first is to find meaning in life. Developmental psychologists and sociologists assert that the knowledge of impending death creates a crisis in which one reviews life in order to integrate one's goals, experiences, and values. This need is met when one can affirm the value of one's life. The failure to find such meaning creates a great sense of despair that one has wasted one's life.

A second spiritual need is to die appropriately. This means dying in a way consistent with one's self-identity. There is no one, right way to die. Not everyone has to "accept" death. Some may fight death bitterly to the end. Others may deny, or even ignore death. Some will want to preserve life until death can be held off no longer while others will want to die while they still maintain some control over their destiny. In short, each person will define an appropriate death differently.

Dying appropriately also means being able to interpret and understand the experience of death. Understanding the meaning of suffering and death is difficult in a society in which pain seems to have no purpose and meaning. Phillipe Aries (1981) in a historical study of death points out how images of the "good death" have been reversed. In the Middle Ages the most feared death was one that was sudden or one that occurred during sleep, for in these cases the dying person had no time for spiritual preparation. In that period, the pain experienced was believed to help compensate for sin; pain on earth diminished the amount of time a sinner would have to spend in Purgatory after death. While a lingering death is more common now, there is often no framework in which to interpret or understand suffering. Now many persons seem to ask for a quick death without pain, even if such a death involves lack of consciousness.

A third spiritual need is a transcendental one: to find hope that extends beyond the grave. Changes in the focus of hope are a hallmark of the terminal phase. Earlier in the illness the person may have expectations (perhaps entirely realistic) of cure, arrest, or remission. In the terminal phase these may still be "desired hopes," but they are no longer considered likely. In other words, the person's hope is focused not so much on physical survival but on the ways that his or her life may continue even after physical death. A young client of mine was diagnosed with cancer. Early in the illness he had hopes of a total recovery. In the terminal phase he began to emphasize his beliefs in an afterlife.

These religious beliefs of an afterlife represent one common way to find what Lifton and Olson (1974) term "symbolic immortality." Perhaps the great interest in near-death experiences and the popularity of Moody's (1975) *Life after Life* arises from recasting a traditional theological mode of belief in an afterlife into a quasi-scientific framework that is more reassuring in a secular age.

There are other modes of symbolic immortality. The biological mode defines immortality by reference to one's progeny. In the creative mode, continuance is found in one's creations whether they are the singular accomplishments of the great or the more mundane contributions of the average. The "eternal nature" and "transcendental" modes, like the theological mode, refer to different belief systems. "Eternal nature" would be a belief that one's remains will, in some way, return to the chain of life. Transcendental beliefs would refer to a wide range of beliefs that assert that death moves one toward union with God or the universe. In the communal mode one's life is seen as part of a larger group; as long as the group survives, each person lives within that community's memory. In the medical mode, a sense of immortality finds expression in the hope that one will live on because parts of one's body, such as the eyes, heart, or kidneys, will live on in others.

In summary, individuals exhibit the same physical, psychological, social, and spiritual needs in any phase of their illness as they have throughout their lives. In the terminal phase certain needs may be sorely threatened, and others accentuated by the nearness of death.

Withdrawal

Something similar can be said for persons' reactions and responses during the terminal phase. People will respond in many, varied ways—cognitively, emotionally, behaviorally, and physically—just as they have during previous crises in their lives. Often that previous history is a good clue as to what reactions and responses to expect in the terminal period.

One common reaction, one often noted by clinicians and

researchers, is that toward the end of the terminal phase many individuals seem to withdraw and disengage from others around them. Many reasons can account for this withdrawal. Some may be physical: individuals' energy levels may be very low, they may be heavily sedated, or they may be drifting in and out of consciousness. Another physical factor that may account for an individual's withdrawal is pain. We have a tendency at times to romanticize the process of dying, but dying is often painful, not only on physical levels, but on psychological, social, and spiritual levels as well.

There may be other factors as well. Individuals may withdraw because they are depressed. Or they may be focusing on meeting their own needs as they prepare for death. For example, focusing on spiritual needs is a time-consuming, reflective, and inward-directed process.

The dying person may withdraw as a natural response to the disengagement and isolation of others. It has long been recognized that medical staff may find interaction with dying persons both more difficult and less rewarding than interaction with the healthy or the merely sick, and therefore withdraw. A similar process may occur in the family as well. Sudnow (1967), in his study of dying patients, describes "social death" as occurring when significant others define the person as dead. In long illnesses, particularly where people are comatose or semicomatose, "social" death often precedes biological death. Even though the person is physically alive, family and friends perceive the individual as dead and begin to withdraw and separate.

Responses like withdrawal can be very upsetting for families and other caregivers. If this withdrawal is evident it is important to assess and understand the factors contributing to it. But it is also important to remember that not all these factors are open to intervention. In some cases families and caregivers have to allow and accept the dying person's withdrawal, finding their individual ways to continue to provide support.

Decisions in the Terminal Phase

When patients move into the terminal phase, they and their families may have to make a number of decisions that can affect not only the quality of the patient's remaining life but also the ways that families adjust following the death. Often the decisions, such as should the patient enter a hospice program and at what point should interventions be ended, are critical.

Should the Person Enter a Hospice Program?

While other phases of life-threatening illness may be experienced within the home and community, the terminal is usually experienced within institutions. Almost 80 percent of people die in hospitals or nursing homes. Many observers have noted that hospitals, because they emphasize intervention, aggressive treatment, and cures, are ill-suited to care for the dying. In these settings dying persons often receive less attention from staff because staff are discomforted by death. Psychosocial needs of the dying often are ignored. In an atmosphere that emphasizes a medical model with cure or control of disease as desired goals, palliative care, and particularly pain control, are sometimes underemphasized. Patients may be subjected to overzealous maintenance or overly aggressive treatment as medical staff seek to ward off death.

Obviously, the reality of how dying persons are handled varies among institutions: Some do a terrible job, others do an excellent job. In any case, numerous variables influence the ways in which institutions both view death and treat their dying clients.

Nonetheless, the observed failure of hospitals to adequately handle death led in the early 1970s to the hospice movement. As a social movement hospice care has had phenomenal success in the United States, growing from a single hospice in 1971 to over 1800 twenty years later.

Hospice in the United States is more of a philosophy than an institution: although hospice care takes place in free-standing hospices and in special hospice units of hospitals and nursing homes, most hospice care is provided at home. Hospice has a philosophy that emphasizes palliative, comfort-oriented care, placing great attention on the management of pain and distress. Hospices have also stressed holistic care that addresses psychological, social, and spiritual needs as well as medical and physical needs. Hospice programs have pioneered a team approach in which physicians, nurses, social workers, counselors, and volunteers join with the dying persons and their families in the determination of care. This is a distinct difference from the physician-centered mode of care generally found in hospitals. Hospices often emphasize maintaining the continuity of the dying person's life by attempting to provide much care at home; institutionalization is generally a last resort. Hospices also recognize a continuing need to provide services, such as bereavement counseling for the family, after the death.

Sometimes people are reluctant to use hospice programs. Many may not have heard of the hospice philosophy or even be aware that hospice programs exist within their community. Sometimes caregivers are reluctant to discuss hospice programs with families since they believe the topic might upset them. Families and dying individuals may believe that entering a hospice program means "giving up." Or they may be troubled by the erroneous belief that once an individual enters a hospie program, he or she will not be able to leave it and will lose eligibility for conventional health care.

As a result of such misinformation, many people who would benefit from a hospice program fail to enter one, or enroll so late in the illness that hospice really cannot provide them with a full range of services. Enrolling a person in hospice when the individual has only a few days to live and is semi- or virtually comatose means that the person cannot draw upon the counseling services and social support that hospice can provide to increase the quality of remaining time.

Hospice programs can be a wonderful resource for a dying person and family. Hospice physicians and nurses often excel at keeping individuals physically comfortable. Counselors, chaplains, and social workers can assist patients and families to meet psychological, spiritual, and social needs. Volunteers can often help with care, providing needed respite for families. Bereavement counseling and support groups can assist families after the death. Many times family members are so impressed with hospice services that some become hospice volunteers themselves.

Physicians, hospitals, and social service agencies can offer referrals to local hospice programs. Many programs are listed in the phone book. Many hospice programs can accept Medicare or other insurance. Information about local hospices can also be obtained through the National Hospice Organization (listed in Appendix 1).

While hospices are a welcome option, they may not be appropriate for every person in the terminal phase. Many hospice programs require the participation of a "primary care giver" such as a spouse, other relative, or friend who can provide ongoing care. Many individuals, particularly elderly ones, may not have such a person. In some cases hospice care will be inappropriate for medical reasons. In other cases it may be inappropriate for psychological reasons: perhaps neither the dying individual nor the family are ready to recognize that there is no hope for cure or significant extension of life. Finally, dying at home may not be appropriate for every family. Certain conditions have to be met if a person is to die at home. Family members have to be willing to nurse their loved one, have basic training in fundamental nursing skills, and have information about the dying process. Special equipment may be required. And both moral support and flexible, multidisciplinary assistance will be needed.

In short, hospice, like any other form of care, may not be appropriate for every family and every person. It is worthwhile, though, to explore with a physician and hospice staff whether hospice would be beneficial in individual cases.

When Should Intervention Cease?

One of the most difficult decisions in the terminal phase involves decisions about whether, when, and perhaps even how to cease medical intervention. Sometimes these struggles are initiated when staff ask families whether or not they should resuscitate a patient. In other cases families may feel that individuals are being kept alive artificially and themselves approach staff about terminating care.

Often these decisions are especially difficult since they are encased in ambiguity. It is interesting to recognize that Western technological society has lost consensus both on when life begins and when life ends. The former issue underlies the debate on abortion and the latter issue underlies debates on passive euthanasia and termination of treatment. Traditional definitions of death based on the cessation of the heart have been made obsolete by technological advances. Even a "living will" does not fully remove such dilemmas, for there may be little medical consensus on its provisions to cease "extraordinary treatment when no reasonable chance of recovery exists." Court cases have yet to clarify what constitutes "extraordinary treatment." The nature of life-threatening illness may make it difficult to interpret "no reasonable chance of recovery." For example, court cases are pending in which family members of persons with AIDS sought to stop medical procedures under that proviso. Physicians, however, have asserted that while AIDS is a terminal condition, a particular opportunistic infection was clearly treatable, and recovery from that infection probable.

While these decisions may cause distress, family crisis, and even legal conflict, they may be mitigated, like any other problems in life-threatening illness, by good communication. Generally, decisions to terminate care are likely to be less problematic when patients, families, and physicians have clearly explored options and expressed their wishes. Actions like a "durable power of attorney," in which a patient designates an individual to make choices on his or her behalf when he or she is no longer capable of doing so, can clearly establish lines of responsibility.

Beyond its value as a statement of the wishes of the patient, a "durable power of attorney" or a "living will" can have value as tools to open family communication. Families can discuss their own level of comfort with the dying person's decision. When individuals have openly stated their intentions, family members are united in their support of his or her wish, and responsibilities are clear, physicians and even courts are far more likely to respect those wishes.

Tasks of the Terminal Phase

In the terminal phase the medical goal has changed from curing illness or prolonging life to providing comfort. The tasks in this phase reflect that transition. Comfort—physicial, psychological, social, and spiritual—is the paramount concern. In order to achieve that comfort, individuals have to face numerous problems that may challenge that goal. Among the tasks they may need assistance with are:

1. Dealing with symptoms, discomfort, plain, and incapacitation

2. Managing health procedures and institutional procedures
3. Managing stress and examining coping
4. Dealing effectively with caregivers
5. Preparing for death and saying good-bye
6. Preserving self-concept
7. Preserving relationships with family and friends
8. Ventilating feelings and fears
9. Finding meaning in life and death

Dealing with Symptoms, Discomfort, Pain, and Incapacitation

The terminal phase is generally characterized by constant physical decline. Dying individuals need to cope with the increasing intrusiveness of symptoms. They are likely to become progressively weaker and more fatigued. Physical deterioration may occur as well, affecting both identity and self-esteem. Throughout this period the dying may become increasingly dependent upon others.

A number of issues may emerge as caregivers assist their patients in dealing with these issues. First and foremost is the issue of pain control. Some degree of pain may be a constant companion throughout the experience of life-threatening illness. Perhaps it was the first symptom that signaled the onset of the illness. Often it is an intermittent or ongoing problem throughout the chronic phase. In the terminal phase, with little activity and diversion, pain can become a pervasive reality. We often tend to ignore and try to avoid this issue. But dying can be painful, and that pain may be more than physical.

Pain is a multifaceted reality, experienced on many levels. On a physical level pain may be experienced both acutely, in sharp intense periods, and/or chronically. Spiritual pain may result as people struggle with the meaning of life and death. The dying suffer the psychological pain of dealing with anxiety and loneliness, and social pain in coping with interpersonal loss. There may be financial pain, as when individuals worry about the financial impact of their illness and death on their families.

Often neglected in the study of pain is what might be called gender pain. This pain is caused when someone is treated not as a person, a man or a woman, but as an object. Any modesty the person may feel is discounted or ignored. One of the best illustrations I know of this occurred on a grand rounds a number of years ago. A group of doctors unannounced and unanticipated surrounded the bed of a seven-year-old leukemia patient. Yanking up the boy's shirt, the head physician stated "Notice the spleen." After each resident had poked around a bit, they all left. There may be other manifestations as well. People may feel the loss of body image, a loss often exacerbated by the neglect of gender-related rituals such as manicures, hair grooming, or shaves. Individuals may also recognize that their sexual needs are ignored. They are no longer allowed to enjoy lovemaking or even cuddling or other forms of intimacy. This too can add to person's pain and subsequent withdrawal.

One wise nurse-practitioner, Phyllis Taylor (1983), defined the ever-present reality of all these forms of pain as "the most critical problem in the terminal phase." According to Taylor, pain sets up a destructive cycle that saps coping resources. Pain, in all its forms, often results in insomnia since pain is most intensely experienced at night when there is little diversion. This leads to greater irritability, causing family and friends to further isolate the person. This isolation increases the patient's depression, lessens coping abilities, and further exacerbates pain. Pain management, therefore, is the basic precondition to maintaining the quality of life and social relationships.

Caregivers may wish to utilize many of the strategies and approaches I described in Chapter 5. Assessing pain and pain behaviors, and employing relaxation techniques, hypnosis, diversion, and imaging are all useful tools that can be utilized in alleviating pain.

But caregivers also have to recognize their role as advocates. They may need to remind medical staff that, now that the terminal phase has been reached, medical goals have changed from curing illness or prolonging life to palliative goals. Caregivers may suggest alternatives such as hospice care where palliative goals are clearly recognized and the dying individual's comfort is the basic priority. Previous medical concerns such as the danger of addiction or the physical risks associated with pain medication, though legitimate during the acute or chronic phases, have less viability in the terminal phase and so may be gently challenged. Today's medicine often does have the technology to offer both pain control and mental clarity. Research has indicated that contingent strategies, that is, offering the terminally ill medication on request, can reduce anxiety and eliminate the need to display pain as antecedent to medication, thereby actually reducing the amount of medication requested.

Once pain is controlled, individuals can address other issues associated with physical decline. Individuals may need information on the meaning and nature of varied symptoms. Is this symptom or disability permanent or might it possibly subside? Is it to be expected? Can it be treated? What other symptoms might be expected? In addressing these cognitive concerns, caregivers need to be sure of the person's real questions. The question "What will occur?" may be a request for information, a cry for reassurance, or a desire to plan. Only when caregivers take time to fully understand the context of questions can they provide answers that are both honest and meet an individual's needs. For example, a man suffering from cancer once rather casually asked me if the back pain was normal. In discussing his concerns he revealed that he had deep fears that this pain might mean the cancer had spread to his spinal cord, evoking fearful images of an uncle's death from a different form of cancer, a death that left his uncle incontinent and paralyzed.

Questions about symptoms may reveal underlying feelings too. Individuals may need to discuss what these symptoms and increased dependency mean to them and what they are feeling. There may be behavioral dimensions as well. They may need to develop ways that they can more effectively cope with new and increasing limitations and incapacitation. Even limited intervention can help maintain dignity and reinforce a small sense of control. One man, for example, facing deteriorating bladder control, was able to develop an "emergency" code on his nurses' button that allowed him a "fighting chance" to get to the bathroom in time. And finally, in the face of continued evidence of physical decline, individuals may wish to review treatment decisions and contingencies such as durable power of attorney, living wills, or decisions not to resuscitate.

Managing Health Procedures and Institutional Procedures

Because much of the terminal phase may be lived within institutions, clients have to cope both with the stresses of institutional life and with sometimes painful institutional procedures. Goffman (1961) has described the varied disconcerting aspects of institutional life, such as the facts that treatment is based on organizational rationality rather than individual choice, institutions control very basic behaviors such as eating, and that all twenty-four hours are spent within a single limited environment. Goffman also notes that these factors can generate a sense of role dispossession and depersonalization. In a hospital, one can be reduced to an object of medical care, losing personhood in the process. One's previous life and position can seem lost. These stresses can be exacerbated in certain units such as intensive care where rules are far more stringent.

The first question caregivers, individuals, and families need to consider is whether the institution is an appropriate place. Alternatives to institutionalization in hospital and nursing homes, such as home care and/or placement in an hospice, may minimize or eliminate many stressful conditions.

Hospice care may be the best possible alternative form of care for both dying persons and their families. Hospice care can often be provided within the comfort of one's own home. When institutionalization is necessary, hospice facilities often strive to provide homelike environments. Hospices emphasize palliative care, and have pioneered and mastered effective approaches to pain control. Hospices have also been sensitive to the reality that physical pain is only one form of distress that clients experience. The interdisciplinary approach of hospices addresses psychological, social, and spiritual needs as well as physical concerns. In addition, hospice volunteers can ease the isolation of patients and families. Hospice bereavement services provide additional support to survivors following a death. However, such placements may not always be desirable or possible.

When such options are not available or useful, other strategies may assist in reducing institutional stress. Caregivers, families, and dying individuals should identify and explore factors that are creating stress. Once these issues are identified, one can develop strategies to cope more effectively with them. In some cases a caregiver can serve as an institutional advocate or assist in empowering ill individuals or their families to create changes. For example, one man found his room stressful, since it overlooked a busy street. His wife was able to assist in getting the room changed. In other situations no easy solution may be possible and caregivers may have to assists individuals in developing more effective ways to adjust to the stress.

Often issues of depersonalization and powerlessness can underlie a person's concerns. Thus empowering individuals and families to deal with these issues, or serving as an extension of the power of the person, serves a twofold function. Not only does it resolve the immediate problem, it also reaffirms an individual's sense of power and control at a time when he or she may feel such control is missing. The individual's concern with control has other implications. It suggests the importance that even minor factors can have in exacerbating stress. For example, one man was very upset with bureaucratic slowness in replacing his broken TV. Staff could not fully appreciate his concern, since his roommate was graciously sharing his TV. However, for the individual in question the failure to replace the TV reinforced his own sense of powerlessness and depersonalization, exacerbating his stress. Caregivers can help to reinforce a sense of control by providing choices whenever possible. Such choices may include scheduling times for treatment, having a role in selecting staff, and deciding on the presence of others in treatment.

Even knocking on an open door returns power to people. I learned this lesson early. In my clinical training I met a successful businesswomen now dying of cancer. Each morning I knocked on her door and asked if I could make an appointment to talk. She would open up her appointment calendar and we would negotiate a time. Personalizing the environment may also mitigate institutional stress. Determining a suitable form of address, allowing personal effects, and allowing modifications of the environment increase comfort and lower the stresses of institutional life.

Managing Stress and Examining Coping

In addition to managing institutional stress, dying individuals have to cope with all the stresses peculiar to dying. Roberts (1988) has pointed out that dying is an insolvable crisis in so far as nothing the individual can do can change the fact of impending death. To Roberts, the crisis of dying can overwhelm a dying individual's coping mechanisms.

Caregivers and family members need to respect and to support each individual's attempt to cope with the crisis of dying. Although individuals' ways of coping may differ, caregivers and families should remember that their major goal in this phase is to maintain comfort.

No individual's methods of coping should be challenged unless they affect the health of others or the dying person's well-being. It is worthwhile for family and caregivers to explore with dying persons ways to reduce any stress they are experiencing. In some cases dying persons may wish to minimize stress by withdrawing from stressful situations. For example, one man dying from cancer decided that he really had to withdraw from his small business. As difficult as that was for him to give up that role, it eliminated a great deal of additional stress. In other situations modifications in the person's environment may eliminate some sources of stress. In one situation the hospital where a young boy was dying from cystic fibrosis relaxed its rules on both the number and ages of visitors.

In still other situations, providing additional psychological, social, and spiritual support or strategies such as diversion and imaging can help the dying person cope with any stress. For example, one dying woman found visits from an unstable sister upsetting. Not wishing to bar her sister's visits totally, she did arrange for other relatives to be present whenever her sister's visited.

While it may be worthwhile for individuals to examine their ways of coping, individuals may not have the energy or time to develop new coping styles. In these cases caregivers should emphasize adapting coping style to the crisis. For example, if someone is responding to a crisis with inappropriate anger, it would make sense to try to direct the response into different channels rather than spending a great deal of time in exploring the roots of that anger. As much as possible, use support, and respect current coping strategies.

One particular stress in the terminal phase arises from the sense that time is running out. Caregiver and family sensitivity to that issue can considerably reduce a dying individual's level of stress. I once read a handout at a hospice conference. The handout listed a variety of comments and requests from dying persons. A second column listed typical responses. A third column listed a suggested response. The requests were things like "I would love to smell a rose" or "I'd enjoy a pepperoni pizza." Typical responses were statements such as "Tomorrow I will pick you a rose" or "Thursday the menu includes pizza." The suggested response was always the same: "Do it now!"

Dealing Effectively with Caregivers

Individuals and families have to deal with numerous caregivers. Throughout the terminal phase they may have to cope with physicians, nurses, therapists, technicians, psychologists, social workers, chaplains, volunteers, and more. All these people will have their own personalities and characteristics. And in many cases patients and families will be forced into interactions in which they have little control, with persons whom, to varying degrees, they may find difficult. Too many, even well-meaning, helpers can overwhelm individuals who have limited resources.

Individuals and families need to honestly and openly share and explore their relationships with varied caregivers. This provides opportunities to consider factors that might facilitate or impede relationships with caregivers, to examine any underlying patterns in relationships, and to identify and solve any problems with difficult relationships. Often such examinations may even provide insights into their own relationships with each other and with other informal caregivers among family and friends. It may assist in identifying personal factors and stereotypes that might affect interaction with caregivers. Family members and ill individuals also have to recognize and explore the possibility that they may be projecting their own unresolved feelings and conflicts on to staff. For example, as an individual slides into a terminal decline, both the family and the dying person can feel tremendous anger. This hostility can be directed toward caregivers. Sometimes one particular caregiver becomes the focus of this anger. One older woman I counseled was able to recognize that her dislike for one particular nurse was a projection of unresolved feelings toward her sister. In another case an African-American man was able to recognize that his negative reaction toward the various nurses and aides was connected to antipathy for West Indians.

In some cases staff may not recognize personal feelings and behaviors that inhibit their reactions to certain individuals. Caregiving staff may need assistance in understanding why their own interpersonal styles are perceived negatively by others. They may need to identify their own hidden agendas, and reaffirm the fact that individuals have their own ways to face impending death, perhaps including defenses, such as denial, that some caregivers find troubling. Naturally, family must interact carefully and gently lest they needlessly complicate their own relationships with these caregivers and exacerbate any existing conflicts between the patient and these caregivers.

There are other things family members can do to build positive relations between the dying individual and staff. It is important to help staff to see the individual as a person rather than simply as a patient. Personal effects of the individual can generate a sense of individuality. One male patient's "grandpa" pajamas were a constant conversation starter with staff. Another simple but effective strategy for families is to fill a small bulletin board with pictures of the individual's family and the individual himself or herself engaging in favored activities. Such simple things often can facilitate interaction and the discovery of common interests shared by the patient and caregiving staff. Moreover, pictures and the like serve as a constant reminder of the personhood of the patient.

Preparing for Death and Saying Good-bye

There is a process of anticipatory bereavement that complements the process of anticipatory grief. In the latter individuals mourn a loss that is anticipated. In the former individuals take objective actions in anticipation of, or in preparation for, that loss.

The dying person often wants to get his or her affairs in order in preparation for death. "Putting one's affairs in order" can mean different things for different people. It may mean arranging financial affairs: making sure papers are in order, that the family is aware of critical details, that final decisions regarding business are carried out. It may involve actions regarding family relationships: the dying person may seek to reconcile with an estranged relative, receive a visit from a loved one who has moved far away, or say good-bye to every member of the extended family. Individuals may wish to make decisions regarding extraordinary treatment or power of attorney. They may wish to plan their own funerals. Or they may take other actions to provide a necessary sense of closure.

Caregivers, both formal and informal, can have vital functions when dying persons approach this task. In some cases they can assist individuals in their work, perhaps by serving as intermediaries. In order cases they can review with the persons the decisions he or she has reached; in cases where decisions may be hastily made or impaired by physical or mental disabilities resulting from the illness, caregivers can help guide the individual to make better decisions. Caregivers can also gently discuss or review with individuals decisions that need to be made, but which the individual is putting off.

The decisions individuals make at this point may be of critical importance since they may affect the individual's spiritual need to die appropriately. Caregivers can help them define what is appropriate for them as well as empower them to control that process as much as possible, and they can interpret their actions and wishes to other family members or staff. For some individuals "dying appropriately" may mean peacefully accepting death. For others it may signify a desperate struggle right up to the very end.

Throughout this period there may be additional moments of crisis and distress, causeed perhaps by the knowledge that there is nothing more to do medically, by new disabilities that presage further dependence, by medical crisis, or by final decline. One man, for example, who described himself as resigned to death, found his equilibrium disturbed when further physical deterioration left him incontinent. He openly wept at this new indignity, complainig that he was destined to leave life as he entered, in an infantlike state of dependence.

In the final phases some individuals may find it important to say goodbye. Other individuals may seem to hold on, perhaps waiting for a particular individual to visit or a significant date to arrive. Some may seem to withdraw. Caregivers may have a role in helping interpret these and other behaviors to family and friends, as well as providing support, referral, and assistance at the time of the death.

Preserving Self-Concept

In the terminal phase self-concept is assaulted in many ways. Physical deterioration resulting from the disease can damage self-image and self-esteem. Such deterioration, often joined with decreased energy levels and increased disability, may lead to withdrawal and disengagement from social roles and relationships. The underlying condition or the fact of impending death can create a sense of stigma, of being different, that can inhibit interaction with others. Erving Goffman (1983) in his book *Stigma* describes this reaction as a "flooding" in which the stigma becomes so overwhelming that it impairs the ability to function in other roles. The dying individual is no longer seen as a wife or husband, a mother or father, a sister or brother, a good neighbor, a teacher, or whatever, but only as someone who is dying. People then become awkward or embarrassed in the dying person's presence, and they withdraw from him or her. A destructive cycle is set in motion in which the terminally ill person, treated as less than human, begins to perceive himself or herself in such a way. This may be particularly evident when severe disfigurement accompanies the illness. Therefore family and caregivers must assist the patient in preserving self-concept.

Caregivers' own treatment of the ill individual will be an important factor in his or her ability to preserve a sense of self. Treating the dying person as normally as possible is essential. Continued emphasis on daily tasks such as grooming and dental care reinforce a sense of personhood. The use and care of articles such as glasses, false teeth, prostheses, or wigs can reinforce aspects of identity. The ill individual still needs to be treated as a man or woman, and his or her privacy and dignity still must be maintained. Touching can be particularly important, for physical contact emphasizes the important reality that illness or nearness to death has not made the person unclean or untouchable. However, ill persons should never be touched or hugged without their permission, for touch may be physically painful or psychologically uncomfortable. Observing individuals' comfort with touch, or asking them whether they are open to touch, can avoid creating such discomfort. Finally, models of care that allow individuals mutual participation in treatment not only reinforce a sense of self but also reinforce coping and decrease medical resistance.

As in the chronic phase, ill individuals have to consider the effects of illness on other roles and relationships. In this ongoing process individuals may need to decide which roles they must let go, which they can maintain, and which can be redefined. And they can explore the effects of those changes on their own sense of self.

Preserving Relationships with Family and Friends

For the reasons discussed in the previous section, relationships with family and friends often deteriorate in tandem with the physical health of the individual during the terminal phase. Because the person is perceived now as dying, family and friends may withdraw, or have problems with knowing how to interact, or become overly protective and paternalistic.

Caregivers can do three things to help individuals to preserve their relationships with family and friends. First, the effects of the illness on relationships should be reviewed. For example, if an individual complains of loneliness, one can examine the degree to which he or she is isolated as well as factors that may be contributing to isolation or to a feeling of loneliness. In some cases the individual may not be isolated at all. For example, a feeling of loneliness may result from a lack of *meaningful* encounters. In one case a women dying of cancer wanted to discuss her feelings and her fears for her family after her death. The family had great difficulty with such communication, often trying to deflect such serious thoughts. As a result she felt increasingly dissatisfied and lonely even though she had a constant stream of visitors.

In other cases loneliness can result from an objective isolation. Causes can vary from the family's disengagement and discomfort to the person's own behaviors, such as intense anger, that may be driving the family away. Once the effects of the illness on relationships are understood, the dying person, the family, and the caregiver can develop approaches to mitigate such effects.

Second, it is important to review family interaction for possible negative behaviors. For instance, family behaviors around meals and eating can be very revealing. Family members may not always recognize that needs change and appetite may be affected by illness and treatment. I have sometimes seen families treat a ninety-year-old man like he was a nine-month-old baby, frantically trying to convince him to eat. In ther cases family members can focus so much on the bright side that the individual's real concerns are ignored. These kinds of behavior illustrate how family members can themselves isolate the ill individual, furthering a sense of stigma, and alienating one another.

Third, counselors and other caregivers can be helpful in enabling families, friends, and individuals to interact more effectively with one another. Dying persons and their families sometimes need to be told that they are misinterpreting signals. In one case a middle-aged man dying of cancer complained to me that his wife was withholding information about the school and behavioral problems of their teenaged son. I discovered that she was reluctant to "dump" more problems on her dying husband, particularly because in the recent past he seemed to balk when these topics came up in conversations. With my assistance they were able to understand their past communication difficulties. The husband recognized his own ambivalence: no the one hand he was the boy's father, but on the other hand there were days when he just couldn't cope with another problem. Husband and wife were able to develop a code that could communicate their intentions. Every day the husband would ask about their son, Sean. When she had had problems with Sean, the wife would answer, "You know Sean." The husband would follow up on days when he felt able. On other days he would simply sigh and say, "That Sean." Moreover, both husband and wife were able to identify alternate sources of support to assit the wife and son. In summary, then, counseling can assist families in recognizing that all human needs remain in force until the very end of life.

Counseling may also include advocacy with hospital staff. In some cases dying persons may need modifications of procedures or space so as to meet these needs and preserve meaningful relationships. One hospital was very sensitive to married couples' needs to preserve sexual intimacy, providing them with the space and privacy they required. However, a counselor did have to advocate for similar private space and time for a homosexual couple.

Ventilating Feelings and Fears

While individuals may experience a wide range of emotions in the terminal phase, anxiety, sadness and depression, and guilt are particularly common in the terminal phase. Pattison (1978) notes that dying persons can have numerous anxieties arising from fear of the unknown, loneliness, sorrow, loss of family and friends, loss of control, suffering and pain, regression, and a variety of other sources. Pattison further suggests that anxiety can be alleviated by the caregiver's supportive presence, a willingness to explore fears in an open and honest way, and a readiness to advocate, when suitable, for more-effective pain management or more control.

Sadness and depression too are common in the terminal phase. Kubler-Ross (1969) notes that this sadness can be reactive, a response to losses already experienced, or preparatory, a response to anticipated losses. While sadness and depression are both common and understandable, caregivers should not assume that sadness and depression should never be treated. When the quality of an individual's life deteriorates, physicians, family counselors, and other caregivers should consider possible talk therapies and/or pharmaceutical approaches.

While sadness and depression may be expressed verbally, particularly in reactive depression, or through disengagement and disinterest, it may also be expressed by means of suicidal comments. Suicidal comments are common in the terminal phase, and they should be taken seriously. Suicide rates are higher among those with terminal illness, and possibly more accepted by others. (See Range and Martin 1990; Saunders and Valente 1987; Shneidman and Fabarow 1957).

When individuals express suicidal thoughts, family should inform caregivers. Caregivers may wish to assess how viable the threat is. Four areas of exploration are often helpful.

1. *Immanence*—How soon does the individual expect to attempt suicide? Is it a future thought or a present plan?
2. *Provocation*—What has occurred to make the suicide viable now? Is the individual experiencing a current crisis or new disability?

3. *Plan*—Does the individual have a plan? How well defined is that plan?
4. *Means*—Are the means to complete the plan available? Can the individual physically carry it off?

Three interventions may prove useful in inhibiting a suicide:

1. The comment "I don't want to live" frequently means, "I don't want to live *like this*." Often defining and alleviating the *"like this"* may forestall suicide.
2. Another approach is to delay and contract. Here the caregiver seeks to have the individual delay the suicide and may enter into a contract by which the individual promises to contact the caregiver or to perform some other specified preventive action prior to any suicidal act.
3. Caregivers and families may seek to "suicide-proof" the environment, removing any obvious sharp implements, limiting the presence of medication, and providing regular observations.

Other feelings too may be found in the terminal phase. For example, guilt may be common. The life-review process may make individuals feel guilty about acts they committed or failed to commit in the past. They may feel responsible, morally or medically, for their deteriorating condition or for their failure to respond to treatment. In such cases caregivers will want to assist individuals in exploring their guilt. Sometimes this exploration will help individuals to develop a sense of resolution. Having explored their guilt, they may now be ready to dismiss it. In other cases different interventions may be necessary. Some people may need to resolve guilt by speaking to an empty chair or by writing a letter. They may need to search their religious traditions to find a sense of forgiveness. They may need to develop and participate in rituals, drawn from religious traditions, that provide a sense of atonement.

While anxiety, sadness and depression, and guilt are common responses in the terminal phase, any emotional response can occur. Whatever the response, caregivers can assist individuals and families in examining these emotions, seeing the ways that these emotions affect their life and relationships, and—when necessary—developing strategies that will help them to cope with their emotions more effectively.

In assisting ill loved ones in coping with these emotional responses, family members should remember both the limited time frame and the overall goal of psychological comfort. With death drawing near there may not be time to fully explore every emotional response. It is unnecessary that the individual effectively resolve all previous conflicts. Rather goal should be to facilitate, to the degree possible, emotional balance and comfort.

In the terminal phase individuals often grieve their own impending deaths. Kubler-Ross (1969) described this process as "automourning" or mourning for self. Fulton and Fulton (1971) described a process of anticipatory grief, noting that persons may mourn losses that are impending as well as those that have already occurred. Dying individuals can anticipate and mourn their own loss. Not only does the dying person have to cope with the loss of self and the threat of nonexistence, he or she must simultaneously deal with the loss of loved ones, because he or she faces in impending death the termination of all relationships. This grief may be expressed as sadness and depression or in other responses typical of grief.

But though this grief is normal and natural, family and friends may discourage its expression. In some cases family and friends continue to deny the inevitability of death, urging the individual to maintain a positive attitude. In other cases the dying person may wish to protect the family, assuming a cheerful demeanor. In such cases counselors and caregivers have a special role in providing a safe and supportive environment where clients can express their reactions to loss.

Finding Meaning in Life and Death

In the face of death it becomes important for many people to understand and interpret not only impending death but the whole life as well. Individuals may be deeply troubled about present suffering and anxious about future pain. In some cases these concerns are primarily issues of medical management and pain control.

Caregivers can assure both ill individuals and their family members that the person can be made comfortable, and, when necessary, serve as advocates. Often, though, the concern is far deeper. Families and individuals may need to struggle with the issue of suffering, wondering why God would put them through such pain or even if they can still believe in God. Both may wish to explore their own religious and philosophical beliefs, so that they can find answers to their questions. Often a sympathetic chaplain or other member of the clergy can be a useful sounding board for this struggle.

As individuals cope with impending loss, they may need to struggle with varied spiritual needs, particularly the need to find hope beyond the grave. This hope may be found in religious, transcendental, or other belief systems. I have seen some people find comfort from "medical immortality" where one finds significance in contributing to medical knowledge by participation in experimental protocols or by contributing healthy body parts that will survive and sustain others. These modes of immortality suggest areas individuals may wish to explore in any spiritual struggle. It also reminds family caregivers of the possible psychological value of participation in experimental protocols or body donations. Nonetheless, such options should only be presented, never pushed, for many individuals may not find such actions desirable or helpful. It is also important to recognize that hope is not always limited to beyond the grave. Even as life ebbs, individuals may still hope for a recovery, or remission. It is not unusual that individuals confront the possibility of death one day and the next day talk about a recovery.

Since dealing with loss and uncertainty has a strong spiritual component, holistic care often involves a sensitivity to spiritual needs. This care is distinct from religious care. Effective spiritual care allows individuals to define their own spirituality and describe their own spiritual needs. This may range from religious observances (such as prayer, rituals, and the like) to secular acts (observing a sunset or reading poems). We also have to remember that every experience, even those that are painful and fearful, provide opportunities for continued personal development and growth. While I do not want to romanticize the experience of dying, we can also err when we view a dying person's life only in terms of the past tense.

Developmental psychologists have long recognized that an awareness of finitude can generate an intense search to find meaning in one's life. This search too may be looked upon as another spiritual need: Individuals facing death often engage in a life-review process. In that process individuals reminisce and review their life, seeking to find significance.

The family and caregivers' role in this process is twofold. First, they should encourage and support such reminiscence. Simple acts, such as asking individuals to talk about themselves and their past, may often be enough to generate a flood of memories. Other actions may also prove useful. Reviewing photographs, whether personal or related to a given time period; listening to music popular during a person's early life; and music; journal writing are good ways to engender such memories. Constructing family trees and genograms; asking about the individual's life; reviewing family treasures; sharing family stories and humor; constructing life peaks-and-valley lines; even making pilgrimages to special places can also encourage life review.

Caregivers and family may also have to help dying persons construct a sense of meaning. Often individuals may need to review the work they have done, the lives they have touched, even the events they have witnessed to gain that sense of significance. For example, one ninety-year-old woman who felt she had not accomplished much in her life was able to take great comfort in the fact that she started her life in the horse-and-buggy era and lived to see man walk on the moon. One key role family members can have is sharing feelings about the part the dying individual had in his or her life, recalling kind acts or the ways in which the dying individual affected them. One friend recalls how reminiscing with his dying dad reminded his father of all the good times that they had shared, thereby resolving the father's concern that he had not spent enough time with his son.

Sometimes the life-review process can uncover regrets or unfinished business. Often this may be subtle. For example, an individual may constantly repeat a certain story. In one case an older man repeatedly talked about his time as a young officer, reviewing a clash of wills with an experienced older officer. I noted that this man seemed to figure prominently in his account and asked him what troubled him about the man and the experience. He then told me a story of how he resented the man's authority and advice. Once, to assert his own control, he ordered his men to attack the enemy in a certain way that ignored the older officer's suggestions. His men fell into a devastating ambush, and he had carried a heavy load of guilt since that time.

Counselors and family members can help the individual achieve a sense of resolution. There may be a number of ways that can happen. In some cases there may still be opportunity for some form of resolving action. For example, there was still time and mutual motivation for a dying man to reconcile with an estranged sister. In other cases individuals may need to be redirected; that is, they should be nudged to look at things differently. One dying teacher, for example, had strong regrets about her own children's modest educational accomplishments. She was able to find success, however, in the impact she had upon her student's lives and the achievements of some of her educational protegé. Finally, in other cases individuals may need to spiritually reinterpret their lives. Every faith and philosophical tradition has a concept of forgiveness, including self-forgiveness. Once individuals express regrets or guilt, others may encourage them to draw upon their spiritual beliefs to find that sense of forgiveness and resolution.

During this life-review process it is important for family members and other caregivers to remember three things. First, the life-review process is a time-consuming, individually directed, interactive process. Simply telling the individual what to believe or how to look at some past event does little good. Family members and caregivers have to learn to listen, to suggest, to discuss. Second, family members have to remember the goal of avoiding psychological conflict. This is not a good time for family members to introduce their own unresolved issues or conflicts. They should find other opportunities for closure. Third, not every individual will experience an intense struggle at the end of life. Some individuals may have a constant sense of purpose and meaning throughout their lives. There is little need, then, at the end to do anything but affirm and reinforce that sense of purpose.

Developmental psychologists recognize that the life-review process can be critical. Individuals who complete that process successfully can die with a sense of integrity rather than a feeling of despair. Contributing positively to this process may not only assist the dying individual but also provide a critical sense of closure and contribution that helps family members in their own grief. One client told me how much he learned from reminiscing with his mother. The time was very special. The memories stayed with him and touched him. He took great comfort that they had this time together.

The Special Problem of the Comatose Person

Even in the period that the individual is comatose communication can still continue. It is unclear when people are comatose how receptive they are to external stimuli. But there is anecdotal evidence that suggests some people may maintain hearing, at least on some level. Caregivers need not neglect comatose persons. Family members, for example, can continue communication. Family should be encouraged to stroke or hold or touch the individual while gently speaking to him or her. This can often be an excellent opportunity for family members to finish any remaining business with the dying person. Two cases illustrate this point. One involved an eighteen-year-old boy who always had a difficult time communicating his feelings to his father. As his father lay comatose, he was able to finally verbalize his love. In another case a wife was able to finally forgive her dying but comatose spouse for the ways that his alcoholism had affected their life and family. In both cases this opportunity to communicate facilitated later grief adjustment.

Family members and other caregivers may also use this period for gentle reassurance or continued rituals. One chaplain used to make a point of visiting comatose individuals on his rounds, stopping at the bedside to hold the person's hand and gently recite a favorite and familiar prayer or psalm.

Sometimes in this period, or even with conscious clients, family or caregivers may want to provide permission to die. Let me offer a dramatic illustration. A chaplain visited a woman who had been comatose but seemingly holding on to life for months. Seeing that she was thrashing in her bed, the chaplain took her hand and recited the Lord's Prayer and the Twenty-Third Psalm, two favorites of hers. She seemed calmed, for the thrashing ceased. The woman and her husband had both been orphans. In fact they had met in an orphanage. They had had one child who was killed in World War II. One of the woman's concerns had been leaving her husband alone. Remembering this concern, the chaplain softly told her that it was alright to let go, to die, because her husband's friends would take care of him. She died that night.

Facing Illness as a Family

Implicit in all the previous chapters is the recognition that any life-threatening illness is always a family illness. These chapters are based on the assumption that family members are intimately involved in the illness. Not only the ill individual but all members of the family will have their lives changed in both subtle and significant ways throughout the course of the illness.

It is important to understand the effects of illness upon each family member and the family as a whole. Only then can families understand the ways in which the experience of a member's illness affects them as well as the ways that they influence any individual's response to the illness.

Throughout this chapter I will use the term "family" in the broadest possible context. I define "family" interactively rather than strictly biologically. Family refers to anyone who is part of a close circle with whom the ill person interacts, shares information, and feels bound to by strong personal, reciprocal, and obligatory ties. Some may define this as the individual's "chosen family" or "intimate network." Such a term encompasses not only lovers, but friends, and perhaps even others such as ex-spouses, all of whom may become participants in the person's struggle with life-threatening illness. In my counseling one of my first tasks is, in fact, to determine who constitutes the person's circle or intimate network or "family."

The Experience of Illness: A Family Perspective

The family involvement with illness often precedes the period of diagnosis. Families may be involved by noticing and assessing symptoms or by suggesting diagnostic tests. They may be consulted as the person begins to decide upon a course of action, choosing, for example, to delay or seek medical help. The ways in which individuals and families interact throughout this prediagnostic phase can be very revealing, for they suggest patterns that persist throughout the illness. In one case a young man concealed his symptoms and doctor's visits from his parents and other family members so as not to worry them needlessly until after he knew what his problem was. This protective pattern continued throughout the illness, inhibiting the ability of others to provide support and causing his family considerable frustration and even resentment.

In the prediagnostic period families may have to cope with considerable anxiety and uncertainty. Their responses may illustrate coping mechanisms that will be utilized throughout the illness. Some may deny symptoms or the implications of these symptoms, while others fear the worse. Family members may experience other emotions as well. Often there may be guilt associated with their fears. It is not unusual for family members to worry about what the illness will mean for the individual and *what it will mean for them.* Such thoughts, when recognized as selfish, will become a source of guilt.

Even at this early prediagnostic phase an element of uncertainty about the future may be introduced. Already there may be subtle alterations in behaviors between individuals and families. Patterns of communication, sexual relationships, and even power may be affected by the threat of illness.

In the diagnostic period families learn what they and the individual struggling with disease must face. This is not to suggest that all uncertainty is now over. Even a diagnosis may still leave considerable uncertainty about treatment, course, and prognosis.

It must also be recognized that ill individuals may make disclosure decisions that inform specific family members in different ways. Some individuals may decide not to divulge full information about the illness to any family members or to tell the whole truth to just a few members of the family, perhaps developing cover stories to present to other members. Often children and adolescents will be given partial or even untrue information. In one case an older man found he had cancer of the prostate gland. He shared that information with two of his three adult children, charging them not to tell his wife or other son. He also selected not to share the information with other relatives or friends; to all others, he was undergoing minor surgery for a benign tumor. He reasoned that he did not wish to worry his wife who had a heart condition or cause his other son to return home after he had just relocated in a distant state to begin a new job. In another case a woman who had breast cancer decided with her husband not to tell their ten-year-old son about her true condition. In such cases there may be a certain logic to one's initial position, but it will often inhibit family communication and support, and cause resentment, anger, and guilt later. We often need to clearly evaluate the implications of disclosure decisions.

During the diagnostic phase families have to face the possible threat of a family member's sustained illness and even death. But they also have to face the personal consequences of this illness. The onset of illness can affect each individual's life. Each family member's career and life plans may have to be changed or postponed. There may be new and additional responsibilities, demands upon time, and financial effects. Family members too may have to make disclosure decisions, choosing whom they will need to tell and where they will seek support. When a mother is seriously ill, parents may have fears that their children's development may be disrupted or impeded. With some diseases, such as AIDS, there may be anxiety about the social consequences and stigma that may result. With other diseases, there may be concerns about the effect of the disease upon the health of other family members. Such concern can exist even when a disease is not infectious. Family members may worry that anxiety and added responsibilities may adversely affect their health or the health of others. In short, the diagnostic phase is a crisis characterized by continued uncertainty and anxiety, affecting in individual ways both the patient and each member of the patient's networks.

It is also a time when family members may begin to experience their own grief about the other member's possible death. Researchers have described a process of "anticipatory grief" where family members react to the threatened or impending loss of someone. This grief may be evidenced in a variety of ways: physical, cognitive, affective, behavioral, and even spiritual. Family members may experience such physical effects of grief as aches, pains, or fatigue. They may find it difficult to concentrate or focus, and will have dreams about the ill member. They may experience a range of emotions including guilt, sadness, depression, or anger. They may be lethargic or overactive, irritable, excitable or apathetic. They may face a spiritual crisis, searching for some meaning behind the health crisis. They may become disenchanted with religion, or, more likely, embrace their faith more fervently, for personal comfort or as a part of an implicit bargain with God. These reactions will be individual and affected by the responses of the ill person, their own personality and coping style, the level of information they possess, educational levels, and degree of social support.

The effects of the diagnosis affect the family as a whole. The whole family system is altered. Relationships with the ill member, including power and sexual relationships, may change. Members may take on new roles vis-à-vis one another. Some may become caregivers, others may take on advocacy roles. Often some family members, especially parents of ill children, will begin to search systematically for information about the disease and treatment options. Generally the crisis of diagnosis is a time when interaction and communication among family members is high. In many families the crisis is perceived as bringing the family together and there is a strong sense of family and social support. For example, sometimes different perspectives, perhaps based upon educational, class, or cultural perspectives between family members may be tolerated or even treasured. In times of family crisis, members may have greater toleration for these differing perspectives. In some families, however, the stress of the crisis may exacerbate tensions, reativating preexisting conflicts, continuing old conflicts, or creating new ones.

While the chronic phase lacks the intense crisis atmosphere of the acute or terminal phase, it is often a very difficult period for family members, particularly those living with and caring for the ill individual. Often the support and solidarity experienced in the crisis of diagnosis ebbs somewhat as the threat of immediate death lessens and other family and friends adjust to the continued realities of their own life. The immediate family, however, has to accommodate new demands, responsibilities, and stresses to their own daily routines. For though they must continue, as may the ill individual, school or work, they have to adjust to the regimen, treatment, and illness as well as modifications in role responsibilities, quality of life, and daily activities and patterns that the illness entails.

A family's financial state is likely to be adversely affected by the primary and secondary costs of illness. Often the demands of the illness as well as any social or financial consequences may curtail social interaction with others. Bluebond-Langner (1987), for example, notes that many siblings of chronically ill children often find their own social lives and friendships adversely affected by their sibling's illness. She describes how siblings live in "houses of chronic sorrow," places uninviting to visit, and how almost all plans become contingent on the health of the ill sibling. While Bluebond-Langner's research centers specifically on the brothers and sisters of dying children, the implications of her findings are broader, capturing many of the difficulties experienced by all those who share homes with those in the chronic phase.

The chronic phase is often a period of continued stress punctuated by points of crisis. The tension generated by the illness manifests itself throughout the entire family. It may be evident in acute bouts of depression, sleeplessness, irritability, fatigue, helplessness, and isolation. It may take its toll on emotional stability, or manifest itself in abuse or neglect. It is not surprising that grief therapists (see Rando, 1983; Sanders, 1983) found evidence suggesting that long periods of chronic illness may create issues that complicate grief even after the person's death.

Beyond the stress, families in the chronic phase are often on an emotional roller coaster, affected by the ill individual's health as well as the reaction and responses of that individual and other family members. Family members may feel anger over the disease and the sick person's demands, over the effects of the disease on their own life and the life of the family, and at the toll the treatment is taking on the individual and the family. They may feel guilty about their feelings of anger as well as their feelings of ambivalence. The sources of this ambivalence may be quite varied. In some cases they may be ambivalent about the individual's continued life under these conditions, both seeking some finality and resolution but fearing death. Even the changes in the ill individual's physical state may cause ambivalence, sometimes by evoking sympathy and repulsion simultaneously. They may be ambivalent about their own caregiver roles. Family members too may have great anxiety about the ill member, their own ability to cope, and their own future.

Denial is a common response in the chronic phase, particularly in its early period or at times when the ill member's health seems stable. Indeed, families may exhibit the same range of physical, affective, cognitive, behavioral, and spiritual reactions that an ill individual experiences.

There are often two significant family issues evident in the chronic phase. The first involves the ill member's treatment regimen. Family members may respond in many ways to a regimen, acting as anything from saboteurs to supporters. Some members can become overprotective, seeking perfectionism, or overcontrol, while other family members may exhibit poor and erratic participation in treatment. Family members' responses to the regimen may also vary during the course of the chronic phase. In the early chronic phase when the individual seems to be doing reasonably well, family responses may range from feelings that the treatment is unnecessary and a burden to an almost magical instance upon adherence, hoping that such adherence will stave off disease. In the later part of this phase, characterized by decline, family responses may again range from hopelessness ("Why bother?") to unrealistic expectations. Caregivers and counselors will need to be sensitive to the ways that family reactions and behaviors facilitate or complicate the ill member's own response to treatment.

As the individual's health deteriorates and the family member moves into the terminal phase, family members begin to cope emotionally and in other ways with the now-expected death and the ever growing burdens of care. While some family members may continue to deny death even in the phase of physical deterioration, most family members will recognize the possibility, if not the probability, of death. They may begin to plan both for the individual's death and for their own life after the loss.

In the terminal phase members of the extended family and the dying individual's network will rally around the dying member and the immediate family. Sometimes this can raise issues and cause resentment between family members. In some cases family members may resent what they view as intrusions. The return of family members who have moved away or who have been alienated can reactivate old or continuing conflicts as well as create new ones. In one case a dying woman made a great fuss over the fact that her son, who lived two hundred miles away, visited the hospital almost every weekend. This caused her daughter, who had been her mother's primary caregiver throughout the chronic period, to feel hurt and resentful, renewing long-held feelings about her mother's preference for her brother.

Throughout the terminal phase family members will cope with a variety of reactions and feelings. There may be a sense of ambivalence and relief that the individual's struggle, and their own, is nearing an end. Guilt, anger, sadness, and depression are common. They may feel awkward in communicating and interacting with the person, unsure of how to behave and react. They may feel drained by increasing responsibilities for the emotional and physical care of the dying person. As the individual deteriorates and begins to disengage and withdraw, family members may feel confused, hurt, and rejected. And family members may feel exhausted by the illness.

Family members may also be conflicted about behavior should the individual become comatose. If the person is hospitalized, family members may feel the continued responsibility to visit, while at the same time feeling useless and awkward. Counselors and caregivers can often be especially helpful at this time in reassuring family that they will be kept informed and in assisting them in making decisions about time and priorities. Counselors may also wish to assist family members in interacting with comatose persons. Often simple acts such as stroking the comatose person or taking part in routine physical care can assuage feelings of uselessness. And this period can be a meaningful opportunity for family members to take leaves and finish any remaining business.

In the closing period of life family may have to make or review a variety of decisions, such as continuing treatment, approving autopsies, or allowing donations of body parts. They may have to begin to consider actions that need be taken after the death, such as funeral arrangements and disposition of property. These discussions too can sometimes create individual stress and tension as well as conflicts between family members.

As the individual moves toward death, families may have a need to be present, participating in a deathwatch. At such points there may be an intense concern for privacy, such that even routine medical monitoring may cause resentment and anger. Families may wish to participate in varied rituals such as Last Rites or Anointing of the Sick. Other families may not desire such rituals. When a priest unilaterally began to administer Last Rites one mother of a dying child was highly disturbed both because she was unwilling to recognize the fact of impending death and because she wanted her local priest, rather than the unknown chaplain, to have that role. At the moment of death families may want uninterrupted privacy. They may appreciate time alone to say good-bye and complete any private ritual of leave-taking. While the client's struggle ends with death, family will still have to cope with their own ongoing grief.

Throughout the entire course of life-threatening illness one needs to be sensitive to the effects of the illness upon the whole family. Families are always trying to maintain a dynamic balance, constantly adjusting to the continued changes brought about both by internal changes such as the growth and development of family members and external, societal pressures. Life-threatening illness with all the extensive financial, interpersonal, social, psychological, and spiritual changes that it brings about can seriously threaten that required balance. This is evident in all phases of the illness, but especially at crisis points such as the diagnosis, the terminal period, and times of pronounced deterioration in health.

It may be evident too in times of recovery. Here the recovery of the person, with consequent resumption and reordering of family roles and expectations, may threaten any tenuous balance that had been achieved. It is not unusual that families may experience tension and ambivalence even in recovery.

Family members may share anxiety about reoccurances, fearing another family trial. They may be reluctant to share or to give up roles that they had assumed during the illness. Each change throughout an individual's illness produces both individual and interpersonal effects. Family members may grieve the losses that these latter changes entail, for they mean the death of the family system as it once was. One mother dying of cancer recognized her own ambivalence when her teenage daughter began to take up the chore of chauffeuring the younger children. She deeply appreciated her daughter's newfound responsibility but also mourned her own loss of mobility and function, and even resented the shared confidences, experiences, and closeness that were developing between her daughter and the two younger siblings.

One has to be particularly sensitive to the effects of an individual's life-threatening illness on children in the home. As I noted earlier, Bluebond-Langner (1978) indicated that siblings of dying children often live in homes of "chronic sorrow" where parents are constantly depressed about their ill child. Life often revolves around the disease, with plans constantly changing contingent upon the illness. Well children often feel isolated and anxious as a result of the illness, distressed by the treatment, and even guilty about their own good health. Their emotional, social, and developmental needs are often subordinated to those of the ill child. In some cases, well children even feel that they are the targets of their ill sibling's anger. These findings probably have application more broadly to any case where children are members of families providing care to those with life-threatening illness.

Professional caregivers can assist families by helping to empower more open and effective parent-child communication; aiding and advocating recognition of the child's needs; and helping families identify additional or alternate sources of support for children. In some cases this may be other family or friends. Often there may be family members or friends who wish to provide help but are uncomfortable or threatened by interaction with the ill member. They may, however, welcome the opportunity to show support by providing help with children. In addition, many agencies provide programs such as camps, support groups, counseling, and recreational and respite services to such children.

Factors Affecting Family Reactions

The previous section outlined some of the ways that family members may be affected by and respond to a member's illness, but family members' reactions are highly individual, influenced by a wide variety of factors. Rando (1984) reminds us that we need to view the family from two perspectives. First, each family is a collection of individuals. Reaction to another member's illness will be affected by a range of individual variables such as personality, coping abilities, age and maturity, gender, relationship with the deceased, intelligence, education, mental and physical health, religion and philosophy of life, fears, knowledge of and experiences with illness and death, and formal and informal supports. Second, the family as a whole has its own unique structure and characteristics. These latter include such factors as the number and personalities of the members of the family; their developmental states; the family's position in the family life cycle; interactional patterns; values, norms, expectations, and beliefs; equality of relationship, flexibility, and communication; patterns of dependence and independence; coping styles and problem-solving abilities; and resources and strengths. The illness will also affect the family's responses in such areas as the meaning the illness has for the family as a whole; the symptoms and manifestations of the illness; the stigma associated with the illness; the stress and strains of the illness and treatment regimen; the timeliness and course of the illness.

Shneidman (1978) and Rando (1984) suggest that a number of factors seem to facilitate a family system's ability to cope more effectively with life-threatening illness. These include:

Knowledge of the symptoms and probable cycle of the illness, and training as to how to provide effective care throughout all phases of illness

The ability to participate in the care of the ill individual, particularly in the terminal phase, since participation allows a sense of control

Open and honest communication, including the openness to discuss feelings within the family and with the ill family member

Flexible families structures that allow members to readjust roles throughout the course of the illness

Positive relationships between family members and effective and compatible patterns of problem solving and coping

Availability of effective informal and formal support systems

Social and economic resources and the absence of other crises and family problems, all of which combine to maximize effective coping

Quality medical care and good relationships and communication between family and medical systems

A philosophical or religious belief system that allows a continued sense of hope and provides an interpretive framework for illness and death.

This list suggests other factors that might complicate a family's adjustment to life-threatening illness. These factors include:

Dysfunctional patterns of family relationships, interaction, communication, and problem solving

Unavailability or ineffectiveness of informal and formal support systems

Stigmatizing diseases that inhibit the family from requesting or receiving assistance

Other familial or individual crises concurrent with the illness

Lack of social or economic resources

Poor-quality medical care and poor communication and interaction with medical caregivers.

These factors indicate family groups that may be at particular risk. Families that include members suffering from feared diseases such as AIDS may have to face stigma that will inhibit support throughout the illness and even after death and that even strain relationships with some members of the caregiving community. Family units that have experienced the fragmentation caused by separation or divorce may also experience special difficulties. For example, a single parent coping with a child with life-threatening disease might well face a lack of financial, social, psychological, emotional, and spiritual support. Similarly, ex-spouses and separated couples may face special problems when one person becomes terminally ill. Here expectations and norms about appropriate behavior, responsibilities, and even feelings are unclear. Prior conflicts may strain relationships with other family members. Similarly, cohabitating heterosexual couples or homosexual lovers may face similar difficulties because these relationships might not be sanctioned by members of the biological family. The lack of a legally recognized tie may create other problems as well, arising from the role of the partner in treatment decisions, insurance questions, and reaching out for support from informal and formal sources. Families with distinctly different cultural or economic backgrounds may have serious problems interacting with and communicating with medical staff. Certainly, families experiencing social and economic deprivation or those with histories characterized by conflict will have special problems in coping with life-threatening illness.

Families are all unique, each with its own "personality." Just as no two individuals will respond in exactly the same ways to a succession of stressors and crises, no two families will deal with the ongoing problems associated with life-threatening illness in the same ways. Counselers must try to discover whatever strengths a family has, and help the family to best utilize these strengths. Counselers should simultaneously try to understand, correct, and otherwise compensate for any weaknesses that might inhibit the family's response to that illness.

Family Tasks throughout the Illness

Families, just like individuals, will have to integrate the experience of a family member's illness into their ongoing life. For throughout the time of the illness the family will continue to function and develop, to cope with all the continuing tasks of life, and to interact with all the issues and needs that existed prior to the diagnosis. Families, just like individuals, will have to cope with a series of tasks throughout all phases of life-threatening illness. And families, again like individuals, will have varying degrees of success coping with the variety of problems they face.

The Prediagnostic Phase

Just as ill individuals find it valuable to understand their experiences during the prediagnostic period, so may families learn by examining the whole family's role in this prediagnostic period. In some cases families may have had a limited or even no role. They may have known little or nothing about the symptoms. If an individual has kept his or her family in the dark, this action could have positive results if it leads the family to reexamine its patterns of communication, lest individuals continue to show patterns of poor communication—perhaps from a desire to protect—that limit their ability to reach out for or to accept family support. Discussing factors that influenced someone to withhold information about illness may help the whole family learn to cope more effectively in future crises.

In other cases family members may have been aware of symptoms, but minimized or dismissed their significance. Sometimes this occurs because family members wanted to reassure the ill member and themselves that nothing was wrong. Again, discussions can help families identify patterns of behavior and help them to understand the ways that these patterns can either hinder or facilitate the ongoing response to serious illness.

Similarly, family members may wish to examine ways that they interacted and either supported or impeded the ill member during the health-seeking phase. Could they share concerns and reach decisions effectively? Did prior conflicts interfere with decision-making processes? Could they provide emotional, social, and other needed forms of support for the ill member and for each other?

The point of such examination is not to renew conflicts but to understand the ways in which the family functioned. Understand that a family can build on its strengths and compensate for weaknesses, as it engages in a family struggle with life-threatening illness.

The Diagnostic Phase

UNDERSTANDING THE DISEASE AND TREATMENT. Within a family system there may be considerable differences in the ways that family members understand the illness and treatment. These differences can result from a variety of factors: cognitive, educational, developmental, and expectational differences between members; access to different information; emotional and cognitive reactions such as denial that may block understanding; and so on. Assuming that the ill individual is willing to disclose information about the illness throughout the family, family members may need assistance to develop a realistic understanding of the disease. Some family members may have very pessimistic views due to misinformation or prior experiences, and therefore will need some positive reinforcement. Others may be overly optimistic. At this phase of the illness, optimistic responses should only be challenged if they seriously impair family functioning, treatment, or the health of others. In one such case a woman whose son was HIV positive denied that her son was ill since he was asymptomatic. She also badgered her daughter-in-law because she refused to continue having sex with her son. Her conduct caused division in the family and impaired her son's participation in treatment. Here was someone whose false optimism required correction so that she could understand the risks of her son's condition.

REALISTICALLY CONSIDERING THE FAMILY'S ABILITIES TO PROVIDE SUPPORT AND IDENTIFYING ADDITIONAL RESOURCES. The time of diagnosis is an appropriate time for family to begin to develop realistic care plans. Diagnosis usually includes an indication of immediate treatment and caregiving needs. Families that are able to effectively plan and meet these immediate needs will have less anxiety about the future and may well develop effective coping strategies that can be applied to subsequent experiences. Families may need to be made aware of various sources of assistance such as social services, specialized services (for example, for children or for the elderly), community services, and illness-related services. Family members should be encouraged to show such information, for individuals will often identify needs based on their knowledge of available services. Caregivers should assist families in identifying needs and evaluating care strategies. If necessary, they should assist families in examining any sources of resistance to utilizing identified help within or outside of the family system. Strategies that distribute tasks throughout a family and/or utilize outside resources are likely to be more effective both in the immediate crisis and in the long run.

DEVELOPING STRATEGIES TO DEAL WITH ISSUES CREATED BY THE ILLNESS. Life-threatening illness creates immediate problems for the family. Among them are:

Disclosure. Once individuals share information about the symptoms and diagnosis, family members have to be concerned about when, what, and how they talk about the disease within and without the immediate family. Should they tell parents, in-laws, children, or friends? Other family members and the ill member may differ in the degree of secrecy or openness they desire. Caregivers can assist by exploring how these decisions will affect each individual. As I stated earlier, sometimes it is best to adopt a policy of limited disclosure: "What information do I need to share with whom, at what point?" Family members need to be advised that information can often spread geometrically. I knew a teenaged girl whose brother had AIDS and who decided to confide the diagnosis to her boyfriend. Within a short time news of her brother's condition had spread throughout the community, creating additional strain on the family. In another case a twenty-two-year-old woman, out of deference to the wishes of her ill father, decided not to share any information with her roommate and confidant. This decision inhibited her own ability to seek critical emotional support. Through counseling she recognized that her friend could be trusted to keep confidences, and she then decided to tell her friend that she was upset because her father was seriously ill. The point I wish to emphasize is that disclosure decisions can have numerous implications and effects, and thus merit careful consideration.

An issue that often arises within family systems concerns disclosing information to children. Adult members frequently wish to protect a child from troubling information and perhaps protect themselves from the child's questioning. Such strategies are often ineffective because children can sense the anxiety and tension around them. It is often more productive to inform children about what is happening, but to present such information in ways consistent with their own experience and developmental level. Again, limited disclosure is often the best policy. Certainly, any changes they observe should be explained truthfully. Children should also be given the *option* of visiting the hospital if they so desire. Prior to any decision children should be fully prepared for what they will experience. Adults should describe the sights, sounds, and smells that children may observe. Whether children visit or not, they should be given other opportunities to show support, perhaps, for example, by sending pictures, making tape recordings, or phoning. Children should also be supported during the visit. After the visit children need the opportunity to discuss their feelings and observations.

Coping with Professionals and Treatment Decisions. While these tasks are really the responsibility of the ill member, family members may still have strong feelings about them. Caregivers may assist families in identifying and exploring their concerns and assessing how these concerns are complicating or facilitating the ill member's reaction to illness. It is critical that family members are comfortable about treatment decisions made at all phases of the illness. Should the ill person die, the grief of family members will be easier if they are not haunted by questions about whether alternate treatment decisions, including choices of hospitals or doctors, should have been made.

Life Contingencies. The diagnosis of life-threatening illness affects all areas of the ill individual's life and of the lives of other members of the family, such as a family member's decision to quit a job. Counselors can help families to identify their options and review the implications of various decisions. Family members may also need help coping with the uncertainty often evident in the acute period. Often emphasizing that any decision made can be tentative reinforces and facilitates that understanding. But families may need to recognize their own ambivalence and anxiety about uncertainty.

ASSISTING FAMILIES IN EXAMINING THEIR OWN COPING STYLES. Both individual family members and the family as a whole may exhibit coping styles and strategies that are functional or dysfunctional. Nathan (1990) identifies four strategies often found in the early phases of the illness:

1. The *direct/action-oriented* approach is a problem-solving mode in which family members make realistic efforts to deal with the disease.
2. The *conscious/normalcy* mode recognizes the reality of the situation but emphasizes continuing to live life as normally as possible.

3. A third pattern is called *denial/suppression*. Here members eny the disease.
4. Finally, an *escapist* strategy seeks to distance one from the illness by escape mechanisms such as substance abuse.

Nathan notes the last strategy is often the least productive adaptation. Families need to examine the ways that they are responding as individuals and as a family, identifying where and when their strategies are effective, evaluating the ways their coping strategies interact, and considering, when necessary, alternate strategies. Caregivers can help by reinforcing, when evident, effective patterns of coping. It is also important, in the early phase, to emphasize that coping strategies need to be continually reevaluated as the circumstances and family needs change.

FACILITATING COMMUNICATION WITHIN FAMILIES AND BETWEEN FAMILIES AND ILL INDIVIDUALS. The last two tasks have explicitly addressed the issue of communication. Throughout the diagnostic period family members may have needs to discuss feelings and fears as well as issues created by the illness. Caregivers can assist the family by assessing barriers to effective communication and developing strategies to improve family communication. A variety of interventions may be utilized to improve communication. In some cases it is useful to ask members to write down their feelings or to develop structured "sharing sessions." Any such intervention should be suggested only after barriers have been identified within the family.

VENTILATING FEELINGS AND FEARS. Families too may need to express their feelings and fears. They may need to explore their ability to discuss their concerns with one another. They need to consider how their reactions facilitate or impair family interactions as well as the response of the ill member. Caregivers may wish to check "feeling rules" or family norms that govern the expression of feelings. Sometimes families can repress such feelings. Counselors can be very useful here, for they have the opportunity to observe and explore any nonverbal behaviors that may be exchanged when feelings are discussed. Counselors can also lead discussions on how family members respond when feelings are displayed.

EXPLORING THE WAYS THAT THE DIAGNOSIS AFFECTS THE ILL PERSON, RELATIONSHIPS WITH THAT PERSON, AND FAMILY LIFE. The diagnosis of life-threatening illness is often a turning point for ill individuals and their families. Life for everyone will now never be the same. Family members need to reflect upon the ways that the diagnosis has affected the ill member. Some members may not recognize that the person's perspectives and reality have been unalterably changed. And they may be confused or resentful about changes in family life created by the onset of disease.

They also may need to examine their own relationship with the ill individual. Both their perception of the ill person and their behavior toward that person may change as a result of the diagnosis. Parents of dying children, for example, sometimes speak of "diminished expectations." When a child is born, parental expectations may be limitless. Beginning with the diagnosis, though, and continuing throughout the illness, expectations can continually change. By the time of the terminal phase, parents may have considerable fears about their child's future. These diminished expectations can exist in any relationship. These changes in perception can also lead to changes in behavior toward the ill member. One woman, for example, was deeply dismayed when her brother was diagnosed with cancer. She perceived the diagnosis as a death sentence and began to withdraw from him. In other cases fear, anxiety, and misinformation may affect relationships with the ill member. In some cases the diagnosis can become the "master status" or the overarching attribute and identity that defines the individual. The person becomes not the parent or the sibling or the spouse but the "disease victim." This can reinforce that role by removing other significant roles from that person.

The Chronic Phase

ASSISTING IN MANAGING SYMPTOMS AND DEALING WITH CHANGES IN THE COURSE OF THE ILLNESS. Family members may need assistance in assessing the effects of the individual's symptom upon themselves and the family. Goffman (1983), in his book

Stigma, describes "the wise," that is, a group of sympathetic others who understand the stigma created by serious illness and can provide empathy and support. In the chronic phase family members may be called upon to assume such roles. Often they can help the ill member by minimizing possibilities for public awareness of symptoms of the disease. For example, the adult children of a woman with heart disease helped their mother to plan walking routes to church and other events that would minimize physical stress. Family members too may help in reevaluating their roles as conditions change throughout the illness.

ASSISTING THE INDIVIDUAL IN ADHERING WITH THE TREATMENT REGIMEN. One of the ill person's basic tasks in the chronic phase involves adhering to the treatment regimen. But this is not solely a task for the ill individual. By necessity, family members usually become involved in the treatment. In some situations, such as those involving a young child or a frail or disoriented adult, family members may have primary responsibility for the treatment regimen. In most treatment regimens family members will have important roles in encouraging or discouraging adherence.

In designing treatment regimens, especially those that mandate family involvement, caregivers will do well to bring the whole family into the process. Often family members can provide valuable insight on issues that might influence adherence. For example, in one case a son questioned the timing of medication on weekends when family schedules were different and activities were likely to interfere with adherence.

Caregivers also have to be careful about assuming that the family member will participate in the regimen. Family members may feel inadequate to the task of acting as "policemen." They may also be very uncomfortable with other possible regimen-related roles. One woman and her adult son were discomforted by the request that he assist his mother in handling her colostomy bags since it violated family norms of modesty. In other situations family members can be overwhelmed by competing demands on their time. Caregivers can assist families by carefully assessing physical and psychological comfort levels in assigning tasks, providing adequate training, and assisting members in developing additional support, both for backup and respite.

Caregivers might also want to monitor the ways that family members and the person undergoing treatment perceive that the family is facilitating or complicating adherence. And they also should be sensitive to the ways that the regimen is affecting relationships within the family.

PREVENTING AND MANAGING HEALTH CRISIS. Throughout the chronic phase ill individuals may experience medical crises. Families, as well as the ill member, should be informed about ways to avoid crises and how to manage them when they do occur. Often rehearsing strategies for handling medical crises can alleviate anxiety and enhance coping. Once a crisis is resolved, families may need an opportunity to review and reflect upon their ways of handling that crisis. Caregivers may need to intervene to assist families with reviewing in a positive manner, such that strategies of scapegoating are avoided, impediments to effective responses are discussed, and alternate approaches developed. Family members may also need to ventilate feelings and fear arising from the crisis.

REDUCING STRESS AND EXAMINING COPING STRATEGIES. Because chronic illness is extraordinarily stressful for all the members of the family system, some or all members of the family system may need stress management. Families should identify sources of stress and ways that stress is manifested and they should examine their own strategies of coping with stress.

Being a family caregiver is extremely stressful. Not only is the person dealing with constant demands to provide care for the person who is ill, but he or she must simultaneously cope with his or her own sense of loss. Family caregivers may experience an intense range of emotions. They may feel anger and resentment at the person who is ill or at other members of the family system who they perceive as being unsupportive or unappreciative. They may feel guilt about their own inability to be "perfect" all the time for the ill individual. They may find it difficult to cope with the demands of providing the full range of physical, emotional, social, and spiritual support the ill individual seems to require.

These family caregivers may find counseling and self-help

groups useful. They may need to learn how to communicate their own needs to other family members.

Family caregivers and other family members may also find it valuable to learn effective stress-reduction strategies. These can include such things as improving problem solving; increasing planning and communication; withdrawing from stressful situations or delegating; examining and modifying unrealistic expectations of self; and employing effective life-style management such as good diet, regular exercise, social support, diversion, relaxation, and meditation.

Primary caretakers especially must find ways to allow themselves respite. For example, one retired daughter who lived near her father became his primary caregiver during his illness. She came near to burning out, but through counseling finally did learn to effectively use her brothers, both of whom worked and lived some distance away. One was able to come on weekends to care for his father, thereby allowing her and her husband a chance to get away to their vacation home. The other brother assumed responsibility for negotiating with hospitals and physicians. By communicating her needs and recognizing the importance of respite, she was able to minimize stress.

In examining the ways families cope, it is important to remember that each family has its own characteristic ways of coping. Recognizing what these characteristic ways are can be the first step toward utilizing discovering strengths to build on and weaknesses to be corrected.

MARSHALLING OUTSIDE SUPPORT AND RESOURCES. Throughout the chronic phase families will need to effectively utilize informal and formal support systems and cope with medical personnel. Effective utilization of such support can enhance adaptation, reduce stress, and minimize a sense of isolation. This support not only provides needed help and respite, it also has a ritual aspect, affirming that all caregivers are part of a larger group, reinforcing the security of the group in a chaotic time. It is not surprising that family caregivers find that the degree of support a family has prior to the death is an important factor in its adjustment to bereavement after the death. Families need to examine their informal support system, assessing how relationships with friends and families have changed throughout the illness, identifying needs and support available from their informal support network, recognizing barriers to the effective utilization of such support, and developing strategies to utilize such support more effectively. One key issue a family needs to consider is what persons are best suited for which tasks. Not every member has the same level of empathy, patience, commitment, skill, time, and so forth. Some may be good persons to help with shopping or with childcare. Others may help negotiate with medical staff. Still others may be good caregivers or listeners.

A similar assessment should be applied to formal support systems. Caregivers should ask medical staff and others about available services. Counselors must sometimes intervene to help families to explore resistance toward utilizing such services. This may be a particularly helpful strategy if the level of patient deterioration becomes so pronounced that placement in a chronic care facility is necessary. In such cases counselors may need to review with families their own attempts to care for the person, identifying in nonjudgmental ways limits to the capacity to maintain care in the force of the patient's escalating needs. They may find it important to explore alternatives to institutionalization. If the counselor foresees institutionalization, it may be helpful to have families begin to consider what circumstances and events may necessitate it. This allows the family opportunity to consider the possibility and to minimize adverse reactions when possibility becomes actuality. Nonetheless, should permanent institutionalization become necessary caregivers may have to assist families in addressing new emotional or interactional issues that may arise.

NORMALIZING LIFE IN THE FACE OF DISEASE. The simple phrase normalizing life conveys one of the more difficult and complex tasks in the chronic phase. It is one that really entails many distinct issues. The first issue is attempting, as much as possible, to normalize the ill member's life. In order for that member to preserve self-concept, he or she will need to be treated by significant others as "normal." Families need to review the ways that the illness is affecting their perception of and interactions with the ill person. The goal for families is to prevent the illness from dominating their relationship with the ill member so that it becomes his or her primary identity or "master status."

It is also critical to recognize that such treatment can impair an individual's adaptation to illness by damaging self-esteem and coping capacity, and by inducing unnecessary dependence. Often the family members' response to the changes caused by the illness will affect their loved one's adaptation. One study, for example, indicated that husbands' attitudes toward wives' mastectomies affected the women's adjustment and adaptation to illness. Thus it is important to continually assess the ways in which the illness itself is affecting interaction with the ill member, the ill member's response to illness, and the general quality of family life. One doctor routinely asked a simple question: "What changes have occurred in your family since the last visit?" Answering this question, whether asked by caregivers or the family itself, can facilitate an ongoing assessment and attune family sensitivities to the continued changes wrought by the illness. Such a review should also include an assessment of the ways that sexual relationships may have changed between the ill member and his or her partner. And it should also consider financial changes and stresses experienced by the family.

The key to this task lies in normalizing family life *as far as possible*. In some cases families will place such a great effort on maintaining the "usual" life of the family that such effort actually undermines family life and hinders the ill member's adaptation to the illness. For example, one family I worked with attempted to maintain their previous activities and made no allowance for their father's illness. This lessened the social support available to the father, and created additional stress and strain for him. Families should inventory aspects of family life, determine which parts of that life are significant enough to be maintained and which parts must be modified or given up because of the illness, and then allow family members to verbalize their own sense of loss over these changes. This last step is particularly important since it is an unfair burden not to allow family members to recognize that the loss of previous activities is a source of concern. It is not selfish for family members to miss the quality of life and personal freedom that existed prior to the illness.

VENTILATING FEELINGS AND FEAR. In any phase of illness ill individuals and families will need to deal with feelings and fears. Counseling can provide a trusting atmosphere where these feelings and fears can safely be discussed and explored. Caregivers can assist family members in developing effective ways to handle such emotions. Throughout this phase family members may need to examine the many losses that they and their family have experienced throughout the course of the illness. These can include loss of activities, losses of health, and losses of family life and life-style. And they may have to grieve about losses that they anticipate, including the death of the ill member. It is not unusual that feelings and fears may change considerably throughout the course of this phase, swinging from optimism to pessimism, depending on the ill member's current condition.

FINDING MEANING IN SUFFERING, CHRONICITY, UNCERTAINTY, AND DECLINE. Just as ill individuals have to cope with finding meaning in sickness and suffering, so too do other family members. Each family member may be in a different place in the spiritual and philosophical journeys. Family members need to respect these differences.

Families and Recovery

Just as individuals may have ongoing needs even in recovery, so too do families. The family may have changed significantly throughout the course of the illness. It may be difficult to readjust to the recovered member when he or she attempts to assume old roles and relationships. Patterns of independence or dependence formed in the illness may be difficult to change. Family members may experience a variety of emotions at recovery. They may feel anxious about reoccurrence or feel very vulnerable and fragile. They may feel angry as a result of unresolved conflicts arising from the behaviors of other members during the course of the crisis. They may be impatient with the recovering member, perhaps feeling that person's recovery is being paced too slowly or too quickly.

In any case, families should periodically discuss how the family is faring throughout the period of recovery. They may need to validate feelings, noting that this phase in the illness process can be a difficult adjustment.

The Terminal Phase

UNDERSTANDING THE PROCESS OF DYING. When an individual reaches the terminal stage, family members may need to be informed about the dying process particular to that disease. What can they expect, in trajectory, symptoms, incapacitation, and pain? They may need training as to the ways they can respond to any medical conditions or crises they may encounter. They may need assistance in understanding and exploring their own feelings now that the goal has changed to palliative care. They may need to be able to interpret varied signs concerning the proximity and actuality of death. Especially if the family is planning to keep the patient at home, they may find it useful to talk with medical staff about what they can expect in this final period.

But the information a family needs at this stage is not solely medical. Family members may need assistance in interpreting the dying person's social and psychological reactions. They may need help in understanding that withdrawal, anger, grief, and sadness are natural responses to the dying process. And family members may need to explore and to discuss with one another their own responses to such behaviors.

COPING WITH CAREGIVERS AND INSTITUTIONS. The terminal phase often means that family members will again have to deal with a new group of caregivers, those who are actively involved in the care of the dying person. In this phase the dying person may very well be institutionalized in a nursing home, hospital, or hospice. This too can create stress for families. As families explore any difficulty or stresses associated with caregivers and institutions they can develop effective strategies to alleviate problems and stress.

EMOTIONALLY RESTRUCTURING RELATIONSHIPS WITH THE DYING PERSON. While the family continues relationships with the dying person, its members must also begin a simultaneous process of emotional preparation for death. This process must be managed carefully. If this preparation does not take place, the grief period will be much more complicated. Family members can often be surprised by death even when they are aware of the prognosis and the death is preceded by obvious decline and hospitalization. If the family withdraws too soon, however, the dying member can become isolated and this may impair subsequent grieving. Formal caregivers can assist this process by exploring with family members their own needs and reactions. When necessary, they can gently test the family members' sense of reality. And, when appropriate, they can encourage family members to meet their own and each other's needs. In one case, for example, a hospice nurse was able to explore with the wife of a dying man her own needs to be involved in the ongoing life activities of her teenaged children. She was able to assist the woman in arranging for alternate care, freeing her to meet those needs.

EFFECTIVELY UTILIZING RESOURCES. At any point in the illness it is important for family members to consider their effectiveness in utilizing resources such as other family members, friends, and formal services (self-help groups, counselors, and other services). Whenever conditions change, it is critical for family members to reassess their needs and to reconsider their utilization of available resources. Again, families may need to be informed about different types of services that may be able to provide assistance. And again, they may need to explore with a counselor any resistance or barriers toward utilizing such assistance. Often in the crisis of the terminal phase, their informal support systems will rally around. This may provide additional aid and support. But family members may also recognize a sense of resentment for a perceived lack of support during earlier phases of the illness.

DEALING WITH THEIR OWN EMOTIONS AND GRIEF. In the terminal phase, as in any phase of illness, family members may experience a range of emotional responses. As family members face the imminent loss of the dying member, they need to inventory the many losses they have already experienced as well as the losses they anticipate. It is also important, especially after a long illness, for family members to understand that their own reactions to the death may be very ambivalent. They should be reassured that wanting the patient's and their own struggle to end while simultaneously wishing the patient could continue to live is a perfectly normal reaction.

UNDERSTANDING THE HUMAN NEEDS OF THE DYING PERSON. Even though an individual is dying, he or she maintains the same human needs that have persisted throughout life. Humor, love, touch, communication, and care are just a sample of these ongoing needs. Often, though, because families facing the terminal phase are so concerned about the issue of death, they can neglect the individual's other needs. Sometimes formal caregivers can be helpful in assisting families to understand their perception of the dying person and to encourage responses that are cognizant of the dying individual's continuing human needs.

MAINTAINING RELATIONSHIPS WITH THE DYING MEMBER AND CONTINUING TO INCORPORATE THE DYING PERSON WITHIN THE FAMILY SYSTEM. In many ways this is an extension of the earlier task. Not only do families need to be cognizant of ongoing human needs, they need to continue to maintain relationships and continue to incorporate the dying person within the family. In the terminal phase the dying person may have limited energy and be bedridden. Often dying individuals are physically removed from the flow of family life, either because they are confined to a sickroom at home or removed to an institution. Moreover, family members may seek to protect the dying person from additional troubles or difficulties, thus withholding information and removing the person from family decisions. Communication too can become increasingly awkward. Family members may be unclear as to what to say.

It is important for families to openly discuss their relationships with the dying member. To the degree that family members are comfortable participating in activities such as the care of the dying person, or reminiscing, they may provide meaningful interaction for the present and they may also mitigate subsequent grief. For example, when one family was encouraged to share the ways that their father had influenced their lives with him, they found these special times both enjoyable while he lived out his last days and helpful when they later mourned his loss. This activity seemed not only to ease their communication but to be significant for their father and facilitate their later grief. Family members can also participate in other ways that are comfortable for them. Some may choose to be involved in personal care, monitoring medication, providing massages, or helping with grooming. Others may be comfortable in social conversation, or reading to a family member, or even watching television together. That too may provide diversion and social support. Still others may find it helpful to pray with the ill person or participate in other religious rituals. Families should also recognize the need to allow the dying individual the freedom to decide whether or not he or she wishes to pursue these activities.

REALISTICALLY PLANNING FOR THE DYING AND DEATH OF THE PERSON. In the terminal phase family members may be faced with a series of difficult decisions. Some may involve actions to be taken during this terminal phase, for example, decisions to seek hospice care, or to sign "Do Not resuscitate" orders, or to terminate treatment. They may need to decide about autopsies or tissue donations. Families may need help in interpreting signs of impending death and in understanding procedures that may take place around the death. This information is critical in any context, but is essential if the individual is at home during his or her final days. Families will need to know whom to call and when. Other decisions may involve issues related to the time of death, for example, funeral plans. Still others may involve decisions about the post-death period such as decisions about work or selling the home.

The very discussion of these topics can support family members' desire and need to plan. Family members can review the effectiveness of their own problem-solving processes. One man, for example, while facing the death of his wife, became aware that his penchant for unilateral decisions complicated relationships with other members of his family. He was able then to incorporate his children in the decision-making process.

PLANNING FOR THE CONTINUATION OF FAMILY LIFE THROUGHOUT THE TERMINAL PHASE AND AFTER THE DEATH. Throughout the terminal phase and even after the death the family continues. But that family will be affected by the dying process and changed after the death. It is important for families to explore the ways that the illness and death affect the family's communication, interaction, and structure. Families will need to consider how these events have influenced the family's goals and plans. And they may need to consider ways in which they will adjust and prevent fragmentation following the death.

FINDING MEANING IN LIFE AND DEATH. Family members as well as the dying individual need to make sense out of the dying person's life and death. Coming to terms with the ways that a person has influenced one's own life, both for good and for bad, is a critical part of grieving and ongoing personal development. When it is possible, that is, when the reflections are positive, sharing such reflections with the person who is ill and with other family members can help each person's search for meaning. When my father had reached a critical point in his own struggle with cancer, our family shared a meal together. We spoke of all the good times we had had, all the gifts he had given us. I do not think that any of us realized all the different facets of his fathering until that moment. Each of us, including my father, developed a better measure of the man.

Negative feelings, though shielded from the dying individual, should not be bottled inside. They should be shared, but probably with a counselor or a confidant. At this point it is unfair to complicate other family members' struggles with meaning by adding to their burdens.

Families do not have to face the crisis of illness alone. There are many resources that can assist families and ill individuals in their struggle. Both Appendix 1 of this book and the recommendations of physicians and other caregivers can be helpful in locating such services.

In summary, families face considerable challenges when one member if ill. They can face these challenges better if they confront them as a family. Standing together as a family means that each family member feels the freedom to discuss concerns openly and to share in solving problems throughout the course of the illness. This open sharing does not mean that every problem can be resolved to everyone's satisfaction. It does mean, however, that if families set up a process whereby each member's concerns are aired and considered, where family and individual needs are viewed and balanced, and where appropriate compromises are made, families will find that they are better able to withstand the stresses of life-threatening illness and be more effective in supporting each other throughout this stressful time. There is a myth that illness always brings families together. Sometimes it does, but other times the illness experience can hopelessly fragment a family. It is not crisis, but the way a family faces that crisis, that knits a family together.

Conclusion

This chapter began by reminding readers that life-threatening illness is a family illness, affecting all the members of a family in varied ways at all phases of the illness. The family also has needs, reactions, and tasks that are similar to those of its ill member. Families that recognize their reactions and needs and utilize their own unique strengths and resources to more effectively cope with the tasks created by the crisis of life-threatening illness may more effectively adjust to the illness and threat of death. And families may find that their own adjustment to any subsequent loss and grief is eased.

Coping with Loss

Throughout life-threatening illness, particularly in the terminal phase, everyone involved may be experiencing grief reactions, both for losses already experienced and for losses that are anticipated. At the time of the death survivors will have to cope with their feelings about this final loss. Not only may family and close friends experience these feelings of grief, all those involved—including professional caregivers—may experience a deep sense of loss. Whoever feels a sense of attachment to the person who has died, whoever's life has been touched by that person, will find that the death will touch him or her. Wherever there is attachment, there is loss. And where there is loss, there is grief.

There is no way that the words I offer here will erase a loss experience. I once spoke to a group for newly bereaved persons. After the group session finished, members handed in their comments. Under "weaknesses" the person wrote, "It didn't bring me back my husband." Whatever I say here cannot restore a lost loved one or end the pain associated with that loss.

But it can help one understand loss. And sometimes understanding loss helps because it makes you feel that you are not so alone—that the feelings and reactions you are experiencing, in your own individual way, are not so strange and isolating. And that understanding can assist in working through the long and painful process of grief.

The Variety of Grief Reactions

Whenever one faces loss, one experiences grief. The responses that one has as one grieves are very unique and individual. Each person responds differently to loss. Indeed, one may even experience different reactions as one faces different kinds of losses. Reactions to grief can include physical reactions, feelings, thoughts, and behaviors.

Sometimes one may feel grief physically. One may experience all types of physical reactions, including headaches, nausea, insomnia, tightness in the chest, exhaustion, menstrual irregularities, loss of appetite, pains, and sensitivity to noise. Sometimes such physical manifestations may have a direct relation to the loss experienced. For example, it is not unusual for mothers who have suffered the loss of their newborn infants to experience pains in their arms, womb, or breasts, other times there may be no evident connection between the type of loss and the physical reaction experienced.

If one experiences physical symptoms following a significant loss, it is important to have those symptoms checked by a physician who understands grief. In many cases those manifestations may be reactions to loss that will diminish as the person begins to resolve grief. For example, one woman experienced tremors and shakes following the sudden death of her husband. Neurological and medical tests found nothing. As she worked with a grief counselor she recognized that she had experienced these shakes in the past in times of great anger. When she began to realize how angry she was about the death of her husband, her tremors ceased.

Even though physical reactions may be manifestations of grief, it is wise to carefully monitor them. Grief is a stressful experience, and stress can adversely affect health. Having reactions checked by an understanding physician, who is aware of the recent loss, can provide peace of mind and promote good physical health.

Many times one experiences grief emotionally. One may experience a wide range of feelings as one faces loss. Anger, for example, is a common and natural reaction to loss. Someone you loved and cared about has been taken away from you. Such a loss can create a deep sense of powerlessness and rage. You may be angry at God, or the universe, for this unfair act. You may be angry at the person who died for leaving you. Sometimes that anger and rage may be turned toward others who care about you, your family and friends. Such anger can isolate you from others at the very time you must need their support.

Another common reaction to loss is guilt. You can experience guilt in many ways. Sometimes you feel guilty because you believe that you may have caused or contributed to the death. Sometimes survivors can be haunted by the "if onlys": "*If only* I had made him stop smoking," "*If only* I helped him lose weight," "*If only* I had urged her to have a breast cancer exam every year." Sometimes survivors feel guilty because they believe they are morally responsible for a death—that God is punishing them for something bad they had done. When I worked as a chaplain in a pediatric cancer ward, I encountered many parents who experienced this kind of guilt. They were haunted by the idea that God was punishing them through their child for some long-ago secret sin. Sometimes you may experience "role" guilt. A person may regret that he or she had not been a better husband, wife, parent, child, friend, nurse, or doctor. You can also experience survivor guilt, a feeling that you should have died instead of the deceased. And you may even feel guilt over grief itself, feeling bad that you are not doing better or concerned and feeling guilty about doing too well.

Survivors may have other feelings as well. Loss can heighten a sense of vulnerability, creating anxiety. One mother whose teenager died during his sleep told me that in the weeks following her son's death she would repeatedly wake up, unable to fall back to sleep until she had checked each of her sleeping children. Sadness too is a common reaction.

Sometimes survivors experience a sense of relief or emancipation. If someone has experienced the suffering and stress associated with a long, slow decline and repeated hospitalizations, he or she may feel relieved that the ordeal is finally over and that the painful burden is lifted. Sometimes, a death can free us from other concerns or fears. Perhaps the inheritance associated with a relative's death has eased financial worries or an early death has relieved fears of a long protracted illness. Such feelings of relief are perfectly natural, even though they may trouble you and cause guilt.

Grief is often full of these feelings. As with many other stressful times in life, dealing with death often incites contradictory and confused emotions simultaneously. Frequently you may experience many feelings—anger, guilt, anxiety, sadness—all at the same time.

Survivors also may have to cope with their thoughts and cognitive reactions as they respond to loss. For example, they may become preoccupied, confused, disoriented, or unable to concentrate. It is not unusual that work, whether it be at home, at school, or in the office, will suffer. You may have a hard time believing the truth of loss, constantly reviewing the events and circumstances in your mind.

Survivors may search for the meaning of the life and death of the deceased. They may try to understand why this person lived as he or she did and died as he or she did. It may become very important for survivors to understand the contributions and purpose of the deceased's life. Sometimes they may idealize the person who died, emphasizing only his or her positive attributes, and ignoring all the flaws. While this is a natural and understandable coping mechanism, it can inhibit the resolution of grief and create problems for others in the family circle who must now compete with that false standard of perfection.

Sometimes you may have a sense of the deceased's presence or even an experience that leaves you believing that you have seen, smelt, heard, or touched the deceased. One mther whose daughter had died recounted how one day she entered her daughter's room and smelled the perfume that she had buried with her young daughter. Many bereaved have reported such experiences. Once assured that these experiences are not unusual or evidence of mental illness, most people find them comforting.

Each experience of loss is as unique as the relationship an individual had with the person who died. The loss of a spouse is different from the loss of a parent, a child, a sibling, or a friend—not necessarily easier or harder to resolve—but different. Rabbi Earl Grollman in a presentation noted that when one loses a parent, one loses a link to the past. When one loses a spouse, one's present is changed. And when a child dies, one's future is altered. It is a point well made. Each loss is different.

Not only is the relationship different in role, but also in quality. Individuals do not have the same relationship with each of their siblings or children. Each relationship is unique and distinctly mourned. Some relationships are more ambivalent than others, that is, they have mixed elements, a combination of things liked about the person and things disliked. Relationships that are highly ambivalent are usually harder to resolve. Some relationships are more dependent. Some are more intense.

The way people die is different too, and that also affects our grieving. Deaths that are very sudden, or those that follow long painful illness, create unique problems for resolving grief. For example, long illnesses can leave survivors feeling very ambivalent about their loss for many reasons. The person with the illness may be physically ravaged, causing those who care about him or her to feel real pain for the pain their loved one is suffering. The strain of illness can be so unbearable for family and friends that when the person finally dies they may feel a sense of relief and ambivalence—wanting the person to survive but wishing that person's agony and their own to end.

Sometimes the circumstances of death can create special issues for survivors. I knew a man who had great difficulty about resolving the loss of his parent, in part because it happened on a day when he was skiing and was unreachable. Sometimes the behaviors of or decisions made by the dying person or other family members may complicate the grief of other survivors. Some may feel the person gave up too soon, others that he or she failed to accept death. Some may question decisions to continue care, others to terminate it. Even professional caregivers, heavily invested in their patient's care, can be troubled. I once counseled some nurses who believed that a patient and his family were wrong to decide to end care. I had to help them realize that their own need to continue care and their own feelings about an appropriate death were different from those of the family.

Grieving can be particularly difficult when losses are disenfranchised (see Doka 1989). Disenfranchised grief is grief that cannot be openly acknowledged, socially shared, or publicly supported. In some cases grief is disenfranchised because others do not recognize the relationship. For example, friends, lovers, ex-spouses, or caregivers can experience deep grief that others do not acknowledge. Grief can be disenfranchised when losses such as perinatal loss go unrecognized. Sometimes certain grievers, such as the very young, the very old, or the developmentally disabled, may not be perceived as capable of grief. Finally, certain types of death such as death by AIDS-related causes can carry such social stigma that survivors are reluctant to share their loss with others. In many cases of disenfranchised grief the grief process is complicated, but the many supports available to other grievers are absent.

Not only are relationships and circumstances different, each individual is different too. Each person has a unique personality and individual ways of coping. Some people are better able to cope than others. And individuals cope with crisis in different ways. Some persons will bury themselves in work, seeking diversion; some will want to talk; others will avoid conversation.

Sometimes aspects of one's background will affect grieving. We all belong to varied ethnic and religious groups, each with its own beliefs and rituals about death. Sometimes these beliefs, and rituals will facilitate grieving. Other times they may complicate it. For example, perhaps one's religious beliefs provide comfort because of the thought that the person is in heaven, or at peace. Different gender roles, male or female, can also affect grieving. Men, for example, may be more reluctant than women to cry, show emotion, or share feelings. Loss can affect us at different points in our development. A twelve-year-old child and a forty-two-year-old adult will have different reactions to the loss of a parent.

Situations may be different as well. It is harder to resolve grief while simultaneously dealing with all kinds of other life crises. It is harder to deal with the stress of grief if one's health is poor. It is harder to cope with loss if friends and family are unavailable or unsupportive.

Grief is a unique individual and time consuming process, it is a long time-consuming one. I have found it helpful to describe grief as a roller coaster, full of ups and downs, highs and lows. Like many roller coasters, the ride tends to be rougher in the beginning, the lows deeper and longer. Also like roller-coasters, the roughest part of the ride may not be at the onset. The period immediately after a death is often a very busy time. There are many details— from funerals to legal actions—to provide diversion. There may be a protective sense of shock now that death has finally occurred. Family and friends cushion the impact of the death. For these reasons, it may take a few months after the loss before grief really grabs hold. The support of others tends to recede just as one begins to understand the full dimensions of the loss. Many people have false expectations about when they should start to feel better, so that as their grieving deepens rather than lessens, they are seriously troubled by their condition. Recognizing that grief tends to increase before it decreases can reassure individuals that they have not regressed.

Holidays, other special days, and the anniversary of the death are usually the lowest times. Such days are heavily invested with memories. It is natural that the pain of loss would be keen at such times. The anniversary of the death too is often a low point. Here the season and weather remind one of the time of loss. Many dates—the anniversary of final hospitalization, the day of the death, the date of the funeral—may have their own depressing significance. Sometimes there are "settlement" reactions as well. Selling a house, receiving a legacy, or signing papers—all can generate a renewed sense of loss. But sometimes these low points occur for no recognizable cause.

It takes time to cope with grief. One serious misperception of grief suggests that people should get over their losses in a relatively short period of time, perhaps a few months, a year at best. The reality of grief is very different. Psychologists and sociologists who have studied grief state that it often takes years to get over a loss. It is normal and natural to experience low points even years after a loss, though hopefully such lows will be less intense and shorter as time goes by.

Grief and the Family

This discussion of the variety of grief reactions may help one to understand why individual members of a family may grieve in different ways. Indeed, I have found that the bereaved are often troubled when they compare their own reactions to those of others in their families. There are a number of reasons for this. First of all, others may have a different experience of loss. Each member of a family has had his or her own special relationship with the deceased, and therefore has a different reaction to his or her death. Second, each member of a family has unique and individual ways of coping. No one reacts to crisis and loss in the same way. For example, one member of a family may wish to visit the grave while another finds such a visit painful. Third, the patterns of grief can differ. One member of a family may respond with deep feelings of guilt while another one bristles with anger. Or perhaps one family member feels low, while for another the cycle of depression begins to lift.

Sometimes these different ways of reacting and responding can create conflicts within families. Sometimes one individual's responses to loss can complicate rather than help another's grief. For example, in one family that had lost a child the father reacted by plunging into work while the mother felt a more intensive need for his presence. In another case a sister was troubled that her brother, whose grief seemed more intense than her own, thereby indicated that he loved their dead mother more than she did.

If the reactions of another are troubling one's own grief, it is sometimes helpful to recognize that one can never really know or feel the unique pain that someone else is experiencing. It also helps to realize that each person does feel and cope differently. These ways of feeling or coping have little to do with the intensity of love for the deceased.

When families face these problems good communication and intelligent compromise are just as important as they are for so many other of life's conflicts. Perhaps one has not communicated one's needs clearly to one another. Or perhaps one has not recognized solutions since one is so burdened by pain. One family, for example, had a huge conflict over whether or not they should have a Christmas tree the first Christmas after the father's death. They eventually decided that instead of a large natural tree, the usual custom, they would have, at least for this year, a small artificial one. In cases where the experiences of grief impede communication and compromise, counseling can often help break the impasse.

What Helps When It Hurts? Resolving Grief

The work of grieving is some of the hardest work an individual has to do. It is hard. Building a relationship with someone takes years of effort. Letting go involves similar effort. Resolving grief, then, is a long complicated process that involves work at a variety of levels—emotional, cognitive, behavioral, and spiritual.

Researchers (Worden 1982; Rando 1984) find it useful to speak of varied tasks that the bereaved complete as they work to resolve loss.

Accepting the Reality of Loss

Often when a death occurs one cannot or does not want to believe it. One feels it is a bad dream. One wants to believe that the deceased will walk through the door and that life will return to the way that it was.

Often the first sign of recovery is the ability to recognize that a loss has occurred. This does not mean that one is ready to emotionally accept the loss or to adjust to life without the dead person. It only means that one intellectually realizes that the loss has occurred, that a person one loved has died.

Funeral rituals are effective in helping to accept that reality. The time devoted to the funeral, the somber break in routines, the rituals themselves—all are vivid reminders that a loss has occurred.

It also helps to talk freely about the deceased. Often one may find oneself repeating the details and circumstances of the death. This too can be healthy, for it can be a way for the reality of that death to seep into our consciousness.

Facing the Emotions of Grief

This task is one of the hardest. Grief, by its very nature, is an emotionally wrenching experience filled with all kinds of vivid and contradictory feelings. In order to resolve grief one has to understand and work through these difficult emotions.

This may involve many things. Again it often helps just to talk, to pour feelings out with someone who can listen uncritically and nonjudgmentally. Because talking about the death with family members may be counterproductive because such talk increases their pain, it often is better to talk with clergy, counselors, or within self-help groups. What is important is to allow oneself an opportunity to ventilate and explore painful emotions.

For example, many times in grief one may be troubled by such uncomfortable emotions as anger. It is important to recognize that these emotions, however uncomfortable and troubling, are normal and natural responses to grief. Once those feelings are recognized, one can then begin to explore them. What makes you feel angry? Is the anger an overreaction? If it is, what else is really troubling you? How will you deal with that anger? There are constructive or destructive ways to respond to that anger. For example, constructive ways include dealing with it physically (by punching a pillow), screaming at an empty chair, fantasizing, crying, or directing that anger in a more appropriate way. For example, mothers, angry that drunken drivers had killed their children, lobbied for stricter laws and law enforcement.

Guilt can also be dealt with in similar ways. Once one recognizes guilt, it can be examined. It is realistic? Sometimes one can hold oneself responsible for all kinds of things that one could never really control. One cannot foreknow all possible consequences of any act nor maintain perfect relationships. Sometimes when one takes the time to examine guilt feelings, one will recognize that the causes of the guilt are illogical or exaggerated.

Other times, however, one may need to do more. One may find it useful to examine one's own religious and philosophical beliefs to find a sense of forgiveness. Or sometimes one may wish to create one's own ritual to expiate any guilt. One widow, for example, feeling guilty over her impatience as she watched her husband's decline from Alzheimer's disease, later found it helpful to volunteer to help persons with Alzheimer's. Her ability to support other spouses and her kindness toward these people allowed her to feel that she was "atoning" for all the anger and impatience she had experienced during her husband's illness.

Often as one deals with these emotions two themes arise. One is ambivalence. One may have a difficult time coping with natural mixed feelings about the deceased. One may be troubled by previous conflicts, hurt by unpleasant memories of that person. It may help to get in touch with this ambivalence by exploring what one liked about that person and what one will miss, as well as what one did not like or will not miss. Coming to terms with that normal ambivalence will help one to better understand these emotional reactions and find effective ways to cope with them.

Another theme comes out concerns unfinished business. Perhaps there is a word unsaid, an act undone. Once one recognizes what is unfinished, one can find ways to complete the act, to bring a sense of closure. Sometimes it may help to imagine that person in the room and then to simply say what needs to be said. Perhaps it can be written in a letter and burned at the graveside. Perhaps a small private ritual may allow that sense of closure. For illustration, one young child felt a deep sense of guilt that he had not told a favorite uncle that he loved him. We talked about all the ways that he had nonverbally showed his love—the way his face lighted up when he saw his uncle, his hugs and his kisses. But he still felt a sense of incompleteness. Finally he decided to dedicate church flowers to his uncle. Delivering those flowers to the grave, he simply stated announced his love. Now that important business was finished.

Adjusting to Life without the Person

One of the most difficult things about grief is learning to live without the beloved person, adjusting to a world in which the deceased is not present. The loss of someone one loves changes one's world completely. One may experience all kinds of other losses as well. One may have lost not only a spouse but a lover, a friend, a gardener, an accountant, and a cook. One may no longer find pleasure in the old habits, in former activities. Even relationships with other family members and friends may change.

Just getting by may seem overwhelming. One's energy levels and coping abilities are challenged just when one is faced with new tasks and responsibilites. A widow or widower, for example, may all of a sudden need to take on a new job, a function that their spouse once did, in the former case for example, balancing the checkbook or seeing to car repairs, and in the latter case, shopping and cooking. Sometimes it helps if one just assesses how much one's life has changed. Often this helps to give one a perspective that keeps one from being overwhelmed by the massive changes one is experiencing.

It also helps to realize the truth: life will be different. One can spend considerable energy trying uselessly to preserve the past. Life after loss is changed life, but we do have some control over that change. Examine those changes in one's life. If one is feeling overwhelmed, prioritize. What are the tasks that need to be done? What is really most important? What can wait? What can be contracted out, that is, assigned to others?

Examine too one's own coping style. How does one deal with change? How can one minimize the stress that change inevitably brings? How well does one cope with that stress?

Because one is experiencing so much change and stress with loss, it is critical not to increase the level of stress already experienced. There are no rules in grief. Each person should do those things that he or she finds most helpful. But if I were to give one rule it would be "Avoid making any significant change in your life for at least six months," Moving, starting a new job, and other similar changes all complicate the levels of stress experienced and isolate a person from natural support groups. If one can avoid such significant changes, do so.

Often loneliness can be one of the hardest aspects of adjustment. One bereaved father told me that he could not get used to "the continued absence of his daughter's presence." That feeling is loneliness. It does not mean necessarily that one is alone, but it does mean that one misses the presence of a particular person.

As with any feelings, it can help to explore the feeling of loneliness. When do I feel lonely? What are the worst times, the worst periods? What can I do about it? One widow found that the most difficult time for her, her worst moment for loneliness, was dinner time. Once she understood that, she was able to reach out to some other widows and arranged to have dinners with them.

Finding Appropriate Ways to Remember the Dead

The end of grief is not the end of memory, but instead the end of memory with great pain. That is important to keep in mind because often one is fearful that once one lets go of pain, one will cease to remember the beloved person.

The resolution of grief involves finding appropriate images and ways to remember the person who died. A person who has touched our lives always remains part of that life.

One can reflect on that person. What are the special memories one has? What did that person's life teach? What aspects of that person's life does one wish to carry on? Sometimes even when those experiences are negative, one can still remember what one learned through that relationship.

One can consider not only how one will remember that person, but when as well. Some individuals develop special ways or times to remember the person who died. They may be as simple as visiting the grave on special days. Or families may develop their own individual ways to remember. One older widower I know tends his wife's tomato garden. Each harvest he distributes the tomatoes to his neighbors, in the process allowing himself an opportunity to reminisce about his dear wife. Another widow whose husband was a teacher administers a small scholarship fund in her husband's memory. Both examples offer healthy ways of remembering, for they acknowledge loss, celebrate the legacy of the dead person, and allow for individuals to continue to grow and develop.

Rebuilding Faith and Philosophical Systems Challenged by Loss

Another problem that one may experience as one grieves is a crisis of faith. For some people, the nature or circumstances of their loss may challenge their very beliefs. They may wonder why they have suffered such a loss. They may feel the world is unfair. They may feel alienated and separated from God.

These feelings too are very normal and natural. Even C. S. Lewis, a great Christian writer, suffered a crisis of faith as he watched his beloved wife die a slow, agonizing death. "Where is God when you need him?," he wrote, "a door slammed in your face." Later he would realize, "It was my own frantic need that slammed that door." Even those without formal religious beliefs may find their philosophies or perspectives challenged by the loss. Perhaps a sense of fairness or justice that was a previous basis of life has now been changed.

If one is experiencing such conflict, it may help to discuss those feelings with a sympathetic clergyperson or counselor. Rabbi Kusher's *Why Do Bad Things Happen to Good People* or C. S. Lewis's *A Grief Observed* may help. It also may help to understand that doubt too is part of the cycle of faith.

Redeveloping an Identity and Reconstructing Life

There comes a point in loss when one has to painfully choose life—a time when one has to recognize that one now has to reconstruct a life after loss. This task is difficult, for so much in life has changed—including oneself.

Every bereaved person is no longer the person he or she once was. Loss has changed those who survive. And while one cannot control the fear of change, one can control the way one changes.

Catherine Sanders, a grief therapist, often asks her clients three key questions as they begin to get ready to explore their options, their alternatives, and find their new selves. First she asks what do you wish to take into your changed life? What are the skills and attributes of the past that you wish to maintain and preserve? What are the skills and characteristics you have developed as you have struggled with loss and now wish to maintain? Then she asks what do you want to leave behind? What baggage from the past needs to be discarded? What feelings—anger, guilt, and the like— yet need to be worked through? Her final question is what do you wish to add? What new skills or characteristics will be essential to continuing development?

All of this takes time. Perhaps the most important thing to stress is that each person should remember that his or her own time for resolving grief is different. Be gentle with oneself. What other people did, when they did it, how they did it, or how long they did it does not mean that you must do the same things or operate on the same schedule. Even the ways in which people recover can differ. A recent study (McClowry, Davies, May, Kwenkamp, and Martinson 1987) of bereaved parents found that these parents resolved grief in different ways. Some "got over it," resuming previous patterns of life or developing new patterns. Others "kept the connection," perhaps by remaining active in groups like Compassionate Friends, because such activities maintained a sense of closeness to the deceased child. Still others felt they had an "empty space" that they needed to fill with diversion and activities. This study reminds us that while the definition of recovery may mean that one has returned to prior levels of functioning, patterns of recovery and the time it takes may differ for each individual.

Getting Help

Throughout the grieving process one may turn to a variety of resources as one copes with loss. Families and friends can provide powerful assistance in this crisis. They can listen and support. They can offer reassurance that despite the loss and throughout your struggle they will still love and care for you. One widow once told about the significant support her best friend provided at her husband's funeral. This friend pressed a key into her hand. "There will be times," she said, "when you cannot bear to face an empty house. Don't worry, my house will always be open to you."

In other situations, though, one may not feel that level of support. Perhaps the pain felt by family is so great that they also are too grief-stricken to be of help. Perhaps friends do not know how to help. They may be waiting for you to communicate needs while you are waiting for them to offer help. Perhaps you are asking for help that they are unable to give. Perhaps you are missing out on the help you need because you are asking the wrong people to do the wrong things. Sometimes friends may just not be available. Perhaps your pain is too powerful. Your loss too threatening.

Seek out family and friends for support. Cherish their help. But when that help is not forthcoming or is insufficient, be willing to seek additional or even complementary help as well.

Outside help can come in many forms. Throughout the past decade numerous self-help books on loss and grief have been published. Some, like Lynne Caine's *Widow,* are first-person accounts of loss. Others, like Therese A. Rando's *Grieving,* are written by psychologists or counselors and offer sage advice. Books can be a valued source of assistance in grief. They can reassure one that one's reactions and responses are normal and natural. They can provide advice and suggestions for resolving problems. And they can also offer hope that one can live beyond loss. In selecting and evaluating books, remember that each person's loss and methods of coping are unique. One may find it helpful to review what another recommends, but each person should do what seems best and comfortable for him or her.

Another source of help may be offered through self-help groups. In some communities, these may deal generally with loss. In other communities, there may be specific self-help groups for widows, parents, or persons who have experienced a specific loss. As with support groups for persons with a disease, groups can provide reassurance, models, and suggestions for problem solving, as well as an opportunity to examine one's own ways of feeling and dealing with loss.

Counseling can also be helpful to anyone, and especially for those who do not have opportunities to share and explore their feelings. Counseling is particularly important for those who are experiencing a very difficult time dealing with loss. For example, if one is experiencing active suicidal thoughts, a desire to hurt others, increased drinking or use of drugs, or is unhappy with the ways in which one is behaving and reacting, it would make sense to seek professional assistance.

Coping with grief can be a very difficult process. Even after a loved one's prolonged illness, gradual decline, and death, it can be hard to let go. Though another's struggle has ended, survivors need to learn how to struggle with their own feeling and reactions to loss. But they need not struggle alone.

The Sensitive Caregiver

A woman institutionalized in a nursing home was praising her nurse, describing her as gentle and warm, caring and considerate. "Of course," the woman added, "I wish I never had the opportunity or need to meet her." This comment expresses the ambivalent way in which caregivers can be perceived as they care for individuals and families struggling with life-threatening illness. They are important, critical allies in the struggle, and are sometimes perceived as having almost magical powers. Caregivers, families, and individuals can forge powerful bonds. Caregivers can become deeply concerned about and involved with their clients. Indeed, occassionally caregivers are the ones who are unable to let go, even when individuals themselves and their families are ready to accept death.

Yet the caregiver role can generate more than a little ambivalence. Sick individuals and their families may have mixed feelings toward their caregivers. Caregivers, after all, are unwelcome reminders of disease. Individuals who are ill, as well as their families, may resent their dependence on caregivers. Certainly, everyone may wish that the circumstances of life had never brought them together.

To function effectively, caregivers will have to demonstrate sensitivity; a sensitivity to the individual is paramount. They will also need to be sensitive to the culture of the individual, whether that culture is defined by ethnicity, life-style, or social class. They will need to be sensitive to the constraints and nature of their own roles. They will need to intervene sensitively and skillfully when appropriate. Caregivers will need to be sensitive to the social context, that is, sensitive to an individual's family, however defined. And finally, if caregivers wish to avoid the awesome emotional costs that can be exacted when one forms a bond with people engaged in a struggle with life and death, they will need to be sensitive themselves.

In all, there eleven sensitivities that the most effective caretakers manifest:

1. A sensitivity to the whole person
2. A sensitivity to the problem of pain and discomfort
3. A sensitivity to honest, open, and mutual communication
4. A sensitivity to the individual's autonomy
5. A sensitivity to the individual's needs
6. A sensitivity to cultural differences
7. A sensitivity to goals
8. A sensitivity to role
9. A sensitivity to families
10. A sensitivity to different age groups and populations
11. A sensitivity to self

This chapter addresses these eleven sensitivities of effective caregiving. It puts these sensitivities at the center of any caregiving role—whether for the physician, the health aide, the counselor, the nurse, the chaplain, or the social worker. I have seen caregivers in a variety of roles taking a special place in an individual's struggle with life-threatening illness. In each case, it was that caretaker's combination of skill and sensitivity that enabled him or her to contribute in a positive mannor in that struggle.

A Sensitivity to the Whole Person

I remember one doctor on grand rounds stopping by the bed of a man who had cancer. As the interns surrounded the bed, the doctor began to lecture. Still lecturing, the doctor and his entourage departed, never having said a single word to the ill man himself. The doctor was highly skilled technically; indeed, on that level he had much to recommend him. But he was seriously flawed as a healer because he saw people as *patients* with various conditions, bad livers or swollen spleens. He was blind to the fact that patients are people: husbands, or wives, fathers or mothers, baseball fans or balletomanes, rose growers or dog fanciers.

The persons one cares for are not just patients but people, living human beings who are struggling with all the concerns of life. Life-threatening illness, at any phase, is more than just a physical or health problem. Life-threatening illness is a multifaceted crisis, one that affects an individual physically, psychologically, socially, financially, and spiritually.

Effective caregiving means maintaining consistent sensitivity to all the dimensions of this crisis. That holistic approach is the heart and strength of the hospice philosophy. But most caregivers do not have the luxury of only taking a holistic approach when a patient has reached the terminal stage of illness. Nor do caregivers always have the luxury of "specializing." Individuals themselves will often choose the person with whom they wish to discuss specific concerns. It is not unusual for a patient to address psychological or spiritual concerns to a nurse, rather than to a psychologist or a chaplain. One woman, for example, reminded her nurse that the chaplain was not available at that moment, 2:00 A.M., but that she needed to talk now. Her nurse was able to listen, provide support, and later provide referral to other caregivers as well.

A holistic approach affirms the reality that life-threatening illness takes place in a context of life. Throughout the time of illness individuals continue to struggle with the same issues and needs that preceded the illness. Naturally, these issues can and will be complicated by the experience of illness. Caregivers who recognize these struggles will not only facilitate an individual's response to illness, but also reaffirm his or her human identity.

A Sensitivity to the Problem of Pain and Discomfort

Pain will be a major focus of attention for individuals experiencing great pain and physical discomfort, leaving them little energy for anything else. Intense pain can exacerbate psychological distress, disrupt social relationships, and intensify spiritual alienation, but none of these issues can be addressed until individuals achieve at least minimal comfort. One of the most important tasks of caregivers is to help individuals who are experiencing pain to achieve a reasonable degree of physical comfort. They may use a number of strategies to accomplish this. In some cases they may serve as patient advocates, reminding doctors and nurses about the pain problems of the individual. In other situations, they may have the ability to directly intervene. They may be able to provide more powerful, or more effective pain medication. They may be able to teach individuals alternative, nonpharmaceutical techniques of pain control such as imagining and visualizations, relaxation techniques, and other behaviorist and cognitive approaches. Such help will not only allow individuals to experience increased comfort and permit them to consider other issues, but it may also assuage anxieties, reaffirm an individual's sense of control, and build trust and rapport. Strategies for pain control will be very much affected by the phase of life-threatening illness. While pain control may have to be subordinated to medical goals during the diagnostic and chronic phases, it should be the major medical goal in the terminal phase.

A Sensitivity to Honest, Open, and Mutual Communication

Earlier, I emphasized the importance of honest and mutual communication. Open communication means responding honestly to an individual's concerns. This is the essence of patient rights and is central to effective caregiving: caregiving cannot be effective in a content characterized by deceit and evasion.

While it is important to provide individuals with information about their illness, it is equally important to do a good job communicating this information. Hogshead (1976) suggests eight principles to employ when delivering "bad news:

1. Keep it simple.
2. Ask yourself, "What does this diagnosis mean to this patient?"
3. Meet on "cool ground" first. Get to know a patient prior to presenting the news.
4. Wait for questions.
5. Do not argue with denial.
6. Ask questions yourself.
7. Do not destroy all hope.

8. Do not say anything that is not true.

These suggestions were addressed primarily to physicians, but they are useful for all caregivers. They remind caregivers of the need to establish a context of open communication.

Avoid cryptic messages that leave people in suspense. It is cruel to say to a person struggling with illness something like "Well, the tests were not as positive as we hoped; we'll talk about it next Tuesday." It is better to say nothing than to provide people with partial information that can only increase their anxieties. Full disclosure, with time alloted for discussion, is the only way to present unsettling news.

There is a nonverbal dimension to open communication as well. The caregiver needs to convey both by the use of space and demeanor as well as words that he or she welcomes communication. Providing privacy, maintaining eye contact, and, when appropriate and acceptable including, reassuring physical contact, facilitate communication. Sitting near an individual rather than behind a desk communicates equality and respect.

An open communication process is both honest and person-centered. Here the caregiver honestly responds to the individual's concerns. For these concerns are cues to what the person is able and willing to hear at any given time. Thus if the individual does not ask about, or does not wish to discuss, prognosis at the time of the diagnosis, it need not be addressed. And if the individual does ask or wish to discuss such issues, they ought to be considered in as tentative and hopeful a manner as honesty allows.

An open communication process tries to accomplish three goals:

1. It lets the individual set the pace and tone.
2. It is reflective. It allows individuals to reflect on their concerns, in effect, to find the answers to their own questions. For example, once a man asked me if I thought he would live to see his new grandchild, expected in about four months. When I asked what he thought, it became an opportunity to share his fear, anxieties, frustrations, and unfinished business. Previous queries to his physician yielded only vaguely hopeful reassurances that showed a reluctance to consider his question.
3. An open communication process provides reassurance that any topic is open to consideration.

Open communication also means trying to understand the individual's perspectives. It is essential that one tries to understand an individual's own biography and perspective. That biography may include items that are part of an individual's history: personal and familial characteristics, religious and spiritual beliefs, cultural perspectives, and informal and formal social support. But it is also critical to understand the individual's perspective on health, illness, treatment, and perhaps, at a later phase, even death.

It is important to understand how an individual became the person he or she is now. To do that, one has to understand the ways in which that individual has struggled with the illness. Often the individual's thoughts and fears about a diagnosis can be very revealing.

Health professionals can be dismissive, or even threatened by, an individual's attempt at self-diagnosis. Yet self-diagnosis can be very informative: it reveals much about the individual's medical sophistication, fears, support systems, and early attempts at detection and treatment. Rather than avoiding the individual's perspective on diagnosis, health professionals should encourage such discussion. Beyond providing insight into the person's basic beliefs, this discussion can convey an attitude of respect and help facilitate a context in which the individual is a full participant in treatment.

This step leads naturally into a larger area of concern, understanding the person's perspective on health, illness, treatment, and death. But understanding that perspective is not easy. While caregivers may or may not differ from individuals in terms of psychological attributes, social attributes, and philosophical ideas, they are certain to differ from them in role and perspective. It has often been noted that doctors are accorded almost mystical prestige in our society. The caregiver brings prestige, knowledge, and authority to the encounter, and the ill individual or family member is clearly dependent. Perspective too is dissimilar. The caregiver is dealing with scientific generalities, but the individual is concerned with a specific life, his or her own. Language too, is different. Scientific language is always tentative and probabilistic: "The chance of X occurring is very remote." But individuals who are struggling with illness speak a more concrete language and seek to hear certainty: "X will never occur," or "X is inevitable." Sometimes these differences can also be complicated by educational, class, and cultural differences also cloud the communication process.

Words may have very dissimilar meanings for caregivers and ill individuals. Each person has a personal construction or meaning of the disease that includes images of the disease as well as ideas about its etiology, treatment, and outcome. Susan Sontag (1988) noted that metaphoric meanings connected to a disease may include connotations of weakness, punishment, and/or inevitable decay and death. A person receiving a diagnosis of AIDS, for example, may perceive the disease as being rapid and horrifying, disfiguring and disorientating. Another individual receiving the same diagnosis may have an image of a long, uncertain struggle, but one that allows interludes of remission and perhaps the opportunity of benefiting from a still-to-be discovered cure.

Perceptions of etiology can also differ. Some may perceive the disease as an unlucky event, others as divine wrath. Given current knowledge that emphasizes life-style factors in disease, it is not unusual for individuals to identify life-style factors that they believe contributed to the disease. But the degree to which someone attributes illness to his or her own behavior, and the feelings he or she has about personal responsibility for illness can differ widely.

People habitually reinterpret the past to make sense of the present. Individual perceptions concerning the etiology of a disease may include numerous segments of biography that the individual believes brought him or her to this moment. And there may be considerable affect, including anger and guilt, in that reconstruction.

Images and theories of treatment may vary as well. Certain individuals with cancer may have a deep fear of surgery because they wrongly believe that once the cancer is exposed to the surgeon's knife it will inevitably grow and spread. Others may have heard horror stories about chemotherapy or fear that radiation will lead to impotence or cause new cancerous growths. Individuals may have self-fulfilling expectations concerning side effects.

People with illness may also have divergent images of outcome. Some may see death as inevitable, others see it as a risk, and still others see it as a remote possibility. They may have images of other outcomes as well. The person who suffers a heart attack may envision a postattack life of near-invalidism. A woman facing a mastectomy may believe her sexual life is over. Individuals may fear that disease will lead to financial impoverishment and familial disintegration.

Even meanings of death can differ. To some, death can be the great enemy, to be fought at all costs. Others may be resigned to death. Some may fear death greatly, others may show less anxiety. Some may see death as an entry to a new form of existence, others as the end of existence.

Images arise from a number of sources. Individuals may have had different experiences with death. Knowledge of the disease may differ. All the variables that affect attitudes—class, culture, age, place in the life cycle, education, religious beliefs, gender, personality—will influence images of illness, treatment, and death.

There may be societal influences as well. Susan Sontag (1978, 1988) suggests that many diseases have a public meaning. She notes that diseases are often used as metaphors—for example, "The cancer of poverty that eats away at the heart of the city." These metaphors influence private meanings of the disease, often complicating responses to a diagnosis. These meanings may change over time, and may not be consistent from society to society. Cancer or leprosy, for example, no longer hold the terror they once held. Historically, even at times when leprosy was prevalent, it was not always perceived in the same manner by different cultures. In some cultures leprosy was greatly feared and lepers ostracized, but in others there was little fear or disgust. AIDS provides a similar example. AIDS is now the most dreaded disease in our society, perhaps because it combines characteristics of other diseases feared throughout history—mysterious origin, disfiguring symptoms, and inevitable fatality—and perhaps because it is passed through blood and semen, bodily fluids that have had universal mystical significance as the fluids of life.

Whatever the roots of patient images caregivers should try to explore the individual's perspective on the disease during the time of diagnosis. Exploration will enable the caregiver to better understand what issues significant for the individual are likely to crop up during the course of the disease and treatment. Every disease creates its own distinct issues, both medically and psychosocially, for care. Colon cancer, and subsequent colostomy, may create deep feelings of shame and possible social isolation. One task of the caregiver in counseling an individual through a life-threatening illness is to understand how the unique issues raised by any given disease and its subsequent treatment will be understood, interpreted, and acted upon by that person.

A second reason for understanding the individual's perspective is guard against what might be called self-fulfilling prophecies. Sudnow (1967), in his book *Passing On,* offers a vivid example of the potency of self-fulfilling prophecies. A man diagnosed with a particularly virulent form of cancer exhibited the normal symptoms and decline characteristic of the disease. Only after his death did the autopsy indicate that the tumor was benign and should not have been life-threatening. In recent years the recognition that a person's perspectives on disease may influence outcome has increased. Certainly, the individual's perspective will influence responses to the disease and treatment. As Rosenbaum (1978, p. 171) states, "The successful long-term treatment of any patient will depend to a great degree on a patient's attitude. If he can strive for and maintain a positive attitude, which means he is willing to fight for his life and believes he can live longer by doing so, he often will respond better to treatment."

Caregivers need to understand and to work through individual's anxieties about treatment. Siegel (1986) claims that "the most important thing [for an ill individual] is to pick a therapy you believe in," and believes that most negative side effects are the result of self-fulfilling prophecies fostered by physicians and patients. Other research (Chandler, 1965) has indicated that individuals who have a strong persentiment of death, that is, a feeling that death can occur at anytime, an attitude often found in heart attack and stroke victims, exhibit higher levels of anxiety, interpersonal difficulties, and acting-out behaviors. While the topic of impact of an individual's perspective on treatment and prognosis needs more extended investigation, it already seems clear that an individual's perspective does play some role on outcome. At the very least, it can be said that individuals who harbor some hope that the disease can be slowed, if not stopped, have a stronger motivation for treatment.

A final issue in reviewing an individual's biography is to understand earlier crises and the ways in which that person coped with these prior crises. Such discussion may provide a good sense of the individual's circumstances as well as his or her perspective. Some may have lived a life characterized by crises while others may have lives that are less tempestuous. Some may define a wide range of events as crises while others are far more selective. A discussion of the responses to these crises also reveals basic coping strategies. These strategies will often be employed throughout the current crises. Becoming aware of them at this early point allows caregivers, individuals, and families opportunities to discuss the ways that their characteristic coping styles both facilitate and complicate adjustment. And it alerts caregivers to the need to explore what may be occurring when these formerly characteristic coping styles are not utilized in the current crises.

A Sensitivity to the Individual's Autonomy

A sensitivity to the individual means respecting that individual's autonomy. The very experience of life-threatening illness thrusts persons into dependent roles. At times in the illness individuals may be physically dependent. Even if they are not always physically dependent, they are dependent for treatment and information from caregivers. Often they may feel that their lives are out of control.

The sensitive caregiver tries to reaffirm that sense of control by offering choices when possible, rather than simply making dictates, or by allowing families and individuals as much control over treatment and daily routine as possible. Sometimes this can be very simple: for example, simply allowing an individual to choose one time slot for treatment from among three or four possible time slots gives him or her a sense of participation in his or her treatment.

Respecting autonomy also means respecting a person's choices. Every individual will make his or her own choices on how to cope with the illness, how to choose appropriate treatments, and—if necessary—and how to face death. These choices may not always be the choices caregivers would make. Someone else's styles of coping may be very different, as may be his or her ways of responding to illness or death. One nurse, for example, was very troubled because a very special elderly patient had no interest in reconciling, prior to his death, with an estranged son. In another situation caregivers were dismayed that an individual chose to discontinue treatment. Caregivers cannot for people to do this or that; all caregivers can do is to help individuals to understand and evaluate their actions. They cannot make choices for others. Shneidman and Farborow's (1978) dictim that "no one has to die in a state of psychoanalytic grace" is wise advice.

A Sensitivity to the Individual's Needs

Having sensitivity to the individual means, of course, having sensitivity for all of that person's needs. Throughout this book I have emphasized the many needs—physical, financial, psychological, social, spiritual—that life-threatening illness creates. I have also stressed the theme that these needs complement, and at times, complicate the health needs of individuals as they continue to try to live their lives. Sensitive caregivers seek to support individuals as they meet those needs.

There is one special point I want to make. Caregivers should be sensitive to the heightened sense of time that individuals with life-threatening illness sometimes experience. There is an exercise I use in my classes in which each student holds a lighted match as he or she relates the most important moments of his or her life. As the match burns down the person's pace sharply quickens. Individuals with life-threatening illness often in a similar way, but throughout their illness, not just in the few moments it takes for a match to burn. Time is the unknown. They feel well today, but tomorrow they may have a relapse. They may have little patience. There is much to do, to experience, and time is unsure. I mentioned in chapter seven a handout given to hospice volunteers on how they might handle dying persons' requests such as a desire for flowers, a need to talk, a wish to taste pizza. The correct response in each incident was "Do it now."

A Sensitivity to Cultural Differences

In the past decade there has been an increasing concern about the challenge posed while providing care to individuals from different cultural backgrounds. (For example. Dillard 1983, Sue and Sue,

1981). That concern arises from the central fact of caregiving that all good care is based on communication. For communication to be effective, both the caregiver and the individual cared for must be able to correctly interpret each other's verbal and nonverbal messages. This process can become very complicated when different cultural groups exhibit different nonverbal and verbal behaviors. It can be especially complicated when linguistic barriers further complicate the process. Even the use of interpreters can complicate interaction for example, interpreters may seek to shield those for whom they interpret, changing the message to make it more palatable.

Counseling culturally different persons can be particularly difficult. The counseling process is rooted in Western and middle-class assumptions, such as the value of individualism and the importance of self-disclosure. Other cultural groups may not share these assumptions and may be mystified and threatened by counseling. Some groups may be uncomfortable with self-disclosure, particularly, with outsiders. Dillard (1983), for example, indicates that many Asian Americans have been taught to mask behavior and avoid eye contact. He also notes that many Asian females may be uncomfortable if left alone with a male. Leong (1986), in a comprehensive review of counseling with Asian Americans, also suggests that Asian Americans may not respond well to unstructured and ambiguous counseling contexts.

Providing care to individuals with life-threatening illness is also complicated by the fact that different cultural groups have different expectations, attitudes, beliefs, behaviors, and values concerning health, illness, pain, and death. Cultural groups may differ on definitions of illness as well as theories of etiology and treatment.

Western medicine often focuses on immediate (for example, virus, bacteria, trauma, and so forth) and underlying (for example, poor sanitation, poor nutrition, weakness due to drug abuse, and so forth) causes, while many other cultural systems will focus on ultimate causes (for example, God's will or sin). Caregivers also should be aware that cultural expectations can influence relationships with caregivers and expectations about the caregiver's role. Hispanics, for example, may expect that a relationship with a caregiver will be personal and marked by trust. Family involvement in care and consultation is expected, especially with elders.

Standards of etiquette and modesty also differ. Hispanics may expect that caregivers will spend time chatting with their clients prior to taking care of business.

In preparing to care for culturally different persons, the caregiver needs to begin with a strong sense of self-awareness. Counselors need to be cognizant of their own values and biases, comfortable with cultural differences, and ready to refer their clients elsewhere if necessary. They may also need to recognize that they may be perceived by some groups as representatives or symbols or a repressive system and thus become targets of anger. Caregivers may have to spend considerable time in developing rapport and trust with members of other groups.

Caregivers should also familiarize themselves with the individual's cultural group. Taking such simple actions as placing culturally relevant magazines in the waiting area can facilitate care. Such an act sends a message to the members of the group that the caregiver is cognizant of and sensitive to their concerns. Sometimes members of that culture may be effective resources. In other cases the caregivers can assume a stance of "enlightened ignorance," asking the individual to inform them about their beliefs, traditions, or behaviors that they are unfamiliar with. Often simple questions, such as "Is there anything that you wish us to know about your culture that can assist our work together?," can be quite revealing. If caregivers have frequent contact with members of other culture groups, they should make the effort to learn more about these cultures, seeking out information about their historical experiences, customs, other components of the culture, and especially cultural factors that might facilitate caregiving and coping with life-threatening illness. Such sensitivity is particularly necessary at the very beginnings of the caregiving process. For even the way one defines or describes a group may affect subsequent development of trust and rapport. Many Hispanic groups, for example, resent the label "Spanish." Many gays resent the term "AIDS victim," preferring the term "person with AIDS" or the acronym "PWA."

In studying a culture, caregivers always have to remember the individual. Many cultures are quite diverse, encompassing many values, traditions, and practices. Individuals may have grown up in families that are blended, that is, in families that draw from a variety of cultures. Individuals may differ in the degree to which they identify with a culture. Some may have a strong cultural identity: they grew up in their country of origin or in a strong ethnic neighborhood, have lived in or returned to such areas, participate in traditional events, take pride in their native culture, and socialize primarily with other members of that culture. Other individuals may be at midpoints in the continuum of cultural identity. And for many others, cultural identification can be remote and distant.

Once a culture is understood, and an individual's level of cultural identification is assessed, caregivers can adapt their methods to that culture and draw on that culture's unique strengths. Dillard (1983), for example, suggests that cognitive approaches may work very well with Asians, as they are compatible with beliefs and behaviors about will power and self-control. Dillard also describes how holistic health approaches work very well with Native Americans since holistic practices are consistent with their beliefs and values. In other situations caregivers may be able to utilize strong family support systems. Even traditional beliefs and folk practitioners may have a role. In one of my cases I counseled a Haitian immigrant being treated for cancer who had a recurring dream she would die on a given date. Conventional counseling did little to change her perspective. At the suggestion of a nurse, I contacted a folk healer from her community. He was able to convince her, after a ritual, that the curse implied by the dream was now removed.

Descriptions of the illness and treatment can sometimes be cast in traditional terms. And cultural rituals too may provide comfort and support in crisis. Ryan (1993) tells of an elderly Chinese-American who was dying and who requested that incense be allowed beside his hospital bed. Participating in this ritual seemed to ease his anxiety.

It is also important to recognize that culture is not defined solely by ethnicity. Culture groups can be defined by a variety of variables such as degree of education, social class, religion, or shared behaviors. Each social class, for example, can be defined as a subgroup within the greater cultural group, with its own shared behaviors, values, and beliefs. Again, caregivers from one class may need special sensitivity in assisting members of other classes. Lower income groups, for example, may be highly suspicious of authority, may be fatalistic and resigned about their condition, and may face a variety of economic and social barriers that complicate their adjustment to illness. They may be isolated from both formal and informal social support. Lower income families may also be coping with many concurrent crises. In addition, they may lack personal physicians, receiving much of their care in emergency rooms, thus limiting any continuity of care. On the other hand, some lower-income people have had to fight so hard to survive that they have a toughness that can be utilized as a significant coping skill. Since many lower income person stress immediate gratification, it might be useful to emphasize the short-term benefits of treatment rather than simply stress long-term effects. Illness will present unique issues to each social class. I once counseled a thirty-five-year-old man from a wealthy and powerful family who was dying from cancer. Although his wealth and connections enabled him to receive the best medical care, including participation in some experimental protocols, he and his spouse became angry and depressed during the terminal phase. They had so much, so enjoyable a life, that death seemed particularly unfair. He was extraordinarily angry and distressed that with all his resources he could not surmount the present crisis as he had so easily surmounted other problems in the past.

Religion too can define cultural groups. Caregivers should be sensitive to the unique religious traditions, practices, rituals, and beliefs of individuals. In one case nurses decided to cheer a patient up by celebrating her birthday. They were unaware that Jehovah Witnesses do not celebrate such occasions.

Even shared behaviors may define a cultural group. The AIDS epidemic has made many caregivers sensitive to gay and drug subcultures. In each subculture responses, feelings, and coping behaviors may differ. Medical treatment and counseling interventions will have to be adapted to that culture. For example, in counseling homosexuals with AIDS or HIV infection, caregivers need to be aware of the importance that sexual expression and experimentation had in the gay subcultural of the 1970s. In designing interventions for IV drug users, caregivers should be sensitive to the often-chaotic life-styles of IV drug users, as well as the fatalism and self-destructive behaviors evident in many IV drug users. Many IV drug users have long tolerated poor health along with addiction and have continually faced the risk of death. In each case, interventions may have to be designed that take into account the unique experiences, behaviors, and issues of each subculture. And both groups may harbor a suspicion of counselors and caregivers.

Finally, caregivers too may face their own unique stresses in working with the culturally different customs and behaviors of different groups. Vachon (1987) offers an illustration of a group of nurses who were discomforted by deathbed rituals of a given ethnic group. Caregivers may find it hard to understand the values, therapies, and rituals of other cultural groups. Caregivers may experience their own bias, fears, and anxieties. For example, many caregivers may be uncomfortable dealing with homosexuals or drug users. Communication difficulties also can frustrate caregivers.

In summation, caregivers have to remember that with any population special issues often arise. The sensitive caregiver should try his or her best to adapt to each individual's cultural heritage, situation, or culture.

A Sensitivity to Goals

Throughout the course of the illness, there may be different goals for treatment. In the acute and chronic phases of the illness the realistic goals may involve saving, or at least significantly prolonging, an individual's life. In the terminal phase the goal is palliative, to provide comfort.

The sensitive caregiver must always be cognizant of these larger treatment goals. Many times the issues that arise in the caregiving and counseling process will be affected by treatment goals. For example, I remember two cases that had a surface similarity. In both cases a hospitalized leukemia patient wanted to attend a significant family event. Given the fragile nature of the individual's health, attendence held considerable health risk. In one case, though, the man was in the initial phases of treatment. There was a realistic hope of significantly prolonging his life and even hope of possible cure. Here the counseling goal was to make him aware of the risk he faced by leaving the hospital, and then, later, to help him find an alternate way of being part of the family occasion. In the second situation the woman was clearly in the terminal phase. While her attendance at the family function held risk, this medical risk was secondary to the tremendous psychological comfort of attending. The treatment goal here was comfort, and my first counseling goal was to help the client understand the risk she faced. When she remained committed to her desire to attend the family function, I changed roles to serve as her advocate and facilitator.

This discussion presumes that treatment goals are shared by all involved caregivers and are realistic. When that assumption is not met, caregivers may have to question implied treatment goals. For example, I once observed a scene between a physician and a nurse. The doctor was reluctant to increase pain medication for his patient, expressing concern about possible addiction and adverse effects upon survival. "But," the nurse reminded her, "I thought we believed the patient would not recover? Isn't our goal now palliative?" This question allowed the care team to openly discuss and clarify treatment goals, and then to deliver care based upon these realistic goals. Sometimes too it is the ill individual or other family members who are unwilling to recognize that treatment goals have shifted. For example, in one case a man was deeply upset and offended by a physician's suggestion that he consider hospice care. For though staff and family recognized he was dying, he unrealistically held to the hope of another remission. In such cases caregivers should tread carefully. An ill person's hopes may be explored, but should be up to that individual to set the pace. A person's sense of hope and his or her defenses ought not be assaulted to obtain unanimity on treatment goals. An individual's hope, it is said, should not expire much before he or she does.

A Sensitivity to Role

Effective caregivers recognize the nature and limits of their roles. Caregivers can struggle for the individual only *with* the help of that individual and his or her family. Primarily caregivers will help individuals and families to identify the issues they are dealing with, explore the dimensions of these issues, and find effective ways to cope with their concerns. Primary caregivers share many things in common with counselors. Many of the processes are still the same. One still needs to establish rapport. Varied approaches may be employed, including cognitive ones, as well as expressive therapies such as art, music, drama, play and dance, or even pet therapies. While the content of caregiving is determined by the individual's needs, and based upon the tasks raised at each phase of illness, communicative skills remain the same. Among the most important of these are:

1. *Open-ended questions* that allow more than a "yes" or "no" answer. These questions encourage the individual to share concerns.
2. *Active listening* which includes:
   a. using silence—so that the individual may fill in space
   b. restating content—allows the counselor to assure others he or she is listening; crystalizes client's comments; checks counselor's perception. Generally, the caregiver paraphrases what was said by the individual
   c. reflecting feelings—here the caregiver reflects on the feelings expressed
   d. summarizing content—similar to restating but with more material
   e. summarizing feelings—synthesis of the individual's effective response.
3. *Interpretation of an individual's nonverbal behaviors*—a tentative interpretation of nonverbal behaviors—for example, "You seem anxious". This is often a good technique to facilitate awareness of or expression of emotion. One has to be careful that one recognizes that the nonverbal behaviors are individually expressed and influenced by culture.
4. *Problem-solving skills*—a broad array of techniques that seek definition and analysis of problems and consideration and evaluation of options.
5. *Empathic statements*—summarizations and interpretation from the individual's perspective that allow the counselor to gently confront underlying issues (for example, noting that "It's difficult to experience such disability. Often it makes you feel a little sorry for yourself.") These interpretations are based on prior content.
6. *Theme identification*—the caregiver identifies underlying themes (difficulty in dealing with loss, for example).
7. *Self-disclosure*—revealing your feelings and reactions to

facilitate the other's sense of being understood. (Note: these should resemble the individual's feelings and be brief enough so as not to change focus from the individual under care.)

8. *Perception check*—attempts to tentatively check the caregiver's perception ("You seem very removed today, are you tired or bored?")

9. *Techniques that try to understand the meaning of client's feelings, behaviors, and attitudes,* such as
a. clarification—simply seeks to facilitate client and counselor's understanding: "Are you angry today?"
b. Confrontation—a delicate technique that must be well timed and sensitive to an individual's receptiveness. Confrontations may point to a person's discrepencies (between verbal statements, between or verbal and nonverbal messages), provide alternate frames of reference, or help individuals understand that they are evading issues or ignoring feedback.
c. Immediacy—the caregiver responds with his reaction and interaction with the person. ("I'm finding it hard to stay tuned. We seem to be rehashing old material. How are you feeling about our interactions?")

10. *Action strategies* such as:
a. desensitization—uses counterconditioning and relaxation techniques to reduce anxiety.
b. contract setting—agreement to modify behavior.
c. social modeling—allows the client opportunity to role-play varied situations with counselor feedback.

11. *Affirmation*—that the individual is valued and likeable. Caregivers should remember that certain approaches such as exhortation, false optimism, or careless phrases ("We will all die sometime") are countertherapeutic, alienating individuals and inhibiting open and effective communication. (Based upon George and Christiani, 1981)

While providing care to individuals with life-threatening illness shares similarities with a variety of counseling and caregiving situation, particularly to crisis contexts, some factors make it unique. Shneidman (1978) has identified a number of factors that make counseling the dying unique. While Shneidman more narrowly stresses counseling the dying and focuses upon the terminal phases, his factors may have broader application in other phases of life-threatening illness. To Shneidman, counseling the dying is different because:

The goals are different. Psychological comfort is the major objective. In such a context, defenses and coping mechanisms are respected and rarely challenged by the caregiver unless these defenses threaten the life of the ill individual or others.

I have already discussed the importance of allowing denial. Individuals are under psychological mandate to "accept" their death. The coping mechanism of denial should not be challenged just because the caregiver or family members are uncomfortable with this attitude. And denial is not the only coping mechanism that must be accepted. I once worked with a young man who was dying of muscular dystrophy. He had constructed a vivid fantasy about the value and significance of his life. This distorted image provided critical psychological comfort. In another counseling context I might have tried to challenge that fantasy and then assist the individual in reconstructing a more authentic identity. Here, though, given the limits of time imposed by his life-threatening illness, I could not take that risk. This young man did not have the time to construct a new sustaining identity. Shneidman comments that "no one needs to die in a state of psychoanalytic grace." His wise words should be a reminder to all caregivers that there is no ideal way for every individual to face his or her own death.

2. *The rules are different.* Shneidman particularly notes that transference can be intense during this phase of illness. To Shneidman, the caregiver can become, and even desire to become, a significant other in the client's life. Thus the caregiver can often play an important role in helping that person validate his or her life or more effectively cope with the illness.

3. *Countertransference can be intense.* Whenever caregivers assist others in facing their mortality, they themselves can be reminded of their own mortality and losses. Fulton (1987) has described the "Stockholm syndrome" and applied it to caregivers. The Stockholm syndrome refers to a common process in hostage-taking in which hostages often identify with their captors. Fulton argues that under extremely stressful situations, close relationships

can be forged quickly. Thus caregivers may identify with the individuals under their care and grieve about their illness and deaths. Caregivers may not recognize their grief, or discuss it with peers, since they believe it violates professional norms of "overinvolvement." They may not receive support from friends who may negate such work-related cases. Their grief, then, though intense and real, can become disenfranchised, that is, neither they nor others around them recognize their real loss and grief.

4. *The process is different.* In counseling individuals with life-threatening illness, particularly as it moves into the terminal phase, one no longer needs to work toward reaching a terminal goal. Death itself provides termination.

5. *The caregiver can be more active.* Generally, caregivers seek to challenge individuals to resolve their own problems and difficulties. Given the frailties of life-threatening illness, and the limits of time, caregivers can take more active roles, serving as advocates and ombudsmen. For example, in one case an individual was reluctant to ask questions of her physician. In another life situation the counselor probably would have tried to help her explore her attitudes toward authority and assist her in developing assertive strategies. Here the counselor served as her advocate.

6. *The person sets the pace.* Weisman (1972) notes that individuals often drift in and out of a confrontation with their own mortality—sometimes denying the illness and approaching death, other times confronting their problems. Counseling strategies should allow individuals to set the agenda and pace. It is not unusual for caregivers to have intense conversations with dying persons about anxieties and fears about illness and death one day that are not even alluded to the next day.

7. *The caregiver must also work with families and other survivors.* Life-threatening illness is a family illness, deeply affecting all others in the family system. Working with families during the illness and after the death is critical.

A Sensitivity to Families

I have emphasized throughout this book that an individual's life-threatening illness always affects the entire family. Sensitive caregiving recognizes the familial context of an illness. Sensitive caregivers understand that individuals may define "family" differently and that family interactions are highly unique, influenced by a variety of factors such as culture.

Caregivers should help families examine the ways in which illness affects them as a family as well as the ways that they are coping with illness.

I have found two models particularly useful in assisting families in coping with life-threatening illness. The first, Herr and Weakland's (1979) model of the family problem-solving process, can be generally applied to many circumstances where families have to assess their own problem-solving process and resolve difficulties. The second, network intervention, can also be a very effective technique that can allow family units to effectively use larger systems, both informal and formal, to resolve particular problems. Both will be outlined here as examples of types of approaches to family counseling that caregivers may find helpful.

Herr and Weakland's (1979) Model

1. *Build rapport and make an initial assessment.*
2. *Define the problem.* The first step after developing rapport and beginning an initial assessment is to clearly define the problem. Herr and Weakland caution that often the "identified problem," that is, the problem that the family recognizes, is not the real problem that families actually need to resolve. For example, the "identified problem" may be that the patient does not take his prescribed medication, while the underlying problem could involve such issues as denial, family power, or control. Ideally, by the end of this stage, Herr and Weakland suggest that the family has defined a problem in a way that avoids both negativism and scapegoating, and recognizes the problem as a family issue rather than solely a personal problem. Instead of, for example, a problem defined as "a family member not pulling their weight," the problem is recaset as "a need to better coordinate and distribute caregiving."
3. *Determine solutions attempted previously.* Herr and Weakland note that many times families have attempted various solutions prior to seeking help. Reviewing these attempts will help one to avoid suggesting already failed solutions, to find solutions

that may have been abandoned prematurely, and to se "solutions" that may have complicated problems. This review can often illuminate family dynamics.

4. *Establish goals.* Once problems have been defined and attempted solutions viewed, families are now ready to set goals. Herr and Weakland emphasize that goals should be both realistic and carefully defined.

5. *Comprehend the family system.* Throughout these first four phases the counselor has observed much about family dynamics. Herr and Weakland suggest that now is an appropriate time for families and caregivers to review the family system and its problem-solving process.

6. *Mobilize the family system.* In this stage caregivers assist families in developing strategies that will allow them to achieve their goals. Herr and Weakland emphasize that interventions and their rationales have to be formed within perspectives the family can identify with and understand.

7. *Achieve a successful termination.* Herr and Weakland point out that the goal of all family counseling is termination, that is, helping family members reach the stage at which they can resolve difficulties by themselves and have learned enough about their own problem-solving process that they should not need further counseling. Herr and Weakland suggest that the counselor at termination should emphasize the family's role in resolving its own problems and help the family to anticipate possible problems that may arise. In the constant crisis context of life-threatening illness, however, caregivers need to recognize that families may need continued contact and help. In such situations a model that allows continued monitoring of the family and provides care mandated by the crisis may be a more suitable approach. Herr and Weakland, though, provide a warning about fostering an overdependence upon the caregiver that impairs the family's coping capacity.

Network Intervention

This technique was originally designed for work with troubled and delinquent youths (see Thorman, 1982). It can sometimes be successfully applied to families coping with life-threatening illness. The goal of the approach is to mobilize a network to resolve a particular problem. This approach can work well when the problem is a tangible one open to a quick fix. While discussing this model, I will refer to a particular case in which network intervention was successfully utilized. In that case a woman residing with her spouse and adult child was in the late chronic phase of cancer. This family had no other children. Since the son worked long hours, the woman's care was mainly in the hands of her retired husband, who provided meals, supervised her medication, and took care of the house. The crisis was caused by the sudden death of the woman's husband from a heart attack.

PREPARATORY PHASE. The decision to use the network model should be made carefully, after an assessment by a caregiver that network intervention has a reasonable chance to succeed. In the preparatory phase a counselor needs to assess the problem and determine the potential viability of the network to resolve the problem. Usually such networks consist of twenty to forty people. The counselor may also need to put together a team to assist this process. After consultation with the family network, a meeting is set up, usually to be held at the home of the ill person over two days. This time from at the home allows the network to reconnect and work together, even in the arranging of such details as meals planning and preparation.

In this case, network intervention was considered viable. The family did have financial resources to pay for some services such as homemaker assistance. The primary problems identified, providing for monitoring and supervision of medication, companionship, and meals, seemed tangible and open to intervention. While the family system was quite small, consisting only of mother and son, the family was deeply involved in a small church that had a pastor and parishioners eager to help. A meeting was set for a Saturday and Sunday afternoon, and about twenty people attended.

STAGES
1. *Retribalization Phase.* In this phase people socialize and reconnect.
2. *Polarization Phase.* Here the family and the team present the problem and the group reviews possible solutions. Team leaders may facilitate the formation of small groups to discuss alterna-

tive solutions. Often sides can form when members commit to a given solution. In this case, one group investigated Meals-on-Wheels and other options such as restaurant delivery to ensure that the ill woman would have her meals while her son worked. Another group considered the possibility that church members could share some responsibility.

3. *Mobilization Phase.* The group begins to consider the tasks needed to find a solution. Often the group recognizes the extent of required commitment and the difficulty of the tasks.

4. *Depression Phase.* The group's initial optimism wanes when its members discover that there is no easy solution to the problem and become discouraged by its scope. Some members may be resentful that their ideas were given a fair hearing. The team helps the group recognize and verbalize their frustration. Now the family may renew its request for help.

5. *Breakthrough Phase.* In response to this request for help, the group recommits, reaches a viable solution, and assigns tasks. In this case the group recognized its limits for providing daily meals, since only ten people were able to commit to regularly delivering a meal. Each of these ten people promised to deliver a casserole-type meal that would provide two days' meals. The son resolved to provide meals on weekends and promised to purchase a microwave oven to make preparation of meals and reheating of casseroles easier. These solutions gave members a sense that all ideas were utilized and it limited the cooks' commitment to one day a month. Other members, here about fifteen in number, agreed to serve as companions to the ill woman, visiting her on days when the cooks would not. A church secretary and another parishioner agreed to serve as coordinators for the whole intervention.

This intervention is just one example of the types of techniques that caregivers may find useful. Other approaches may have similar value. The basic point is that caregivers will need to develop both a sensitivity to the needs of the family as well as appropriate interventions to assist families as they cope with life-threatening illness.

Sensitivity to Different Age Groups and Populations

Earlier I discussed the ways that life-threatening illness is different for people at different phases in the life cycle because developmental issues can often complicate responses to life-threatening illness. Sensitive caregivers will recognize the unique issues that arise at any point in the life cycle. They will also recognize that populations that are developmentally impaired may have special difficulties in responding to the crisis of life-threatening illness. This section emphasizes the particular problem of three groups: children and adolescents, the developmentally disabled, and the elderly.

Working with Children and Adolescents

Counseling children and adolescents with life-threatening illness can be very difficult. Caregivers may find themselves emotionally drawn to the ill child and greatly affected by the child's illness and death. Even beyond such intense emotional involvement, counseling children and adolescents creates other difficulties that complicate the counseling process.

One of the first complications is that caregiver-child relationships are always triadic. Caregivers must simultaneously deal with the child and the parents or guardians of that child. Since the needs of the child and the needs of the parents are not always identical, this can impair trust. Young clients may be reluctant to confide in their caregivers because they are unsure of how much the caregiver can be trusted.

Early in their work with children and adolescents caregivers should confront this issue. Caregivers can affirm that the child's confidences will be respected. Depending on the needs of the parents or the child, caregivers can indicate that they will periodically talk with the parents. But in each case the caregivers and the child together should discuss problems, develop a plan, agree about what will be reported to the parents. The one possible exception, caregivers may forewarn the child, is when the child is engaged in actions that endanger his or her life or the life of others, for in such a case caregivers are compelled to speak with the parents. Caregivers should make parents equally aware of this arrangement.

Another issue that often may be a significant one between parents and children involves communication and truthfulness. Many parents take a protective approach toward communication in which they attempt to shield the child from the nature or implications of the illness. Caregivers need to respect these strategies, but they also need to help parents evaluate the implications of such strategies. Often these strategies are not effective since children have access to a wide range of information about the condition: internal health cues; external treatment cues; information from books, TV, and from videos; input from ill peers; and more. Previous studies (Bluebond-Langner, 1978; Doka, 1982.) indicate that regardless of parental disclosure decisions, children often know the nature and seriousness of their conditions. Such strategies can be costly, for they can impair trust and at a critical time in the parent-child relationship, and they may also complicate compliance with medical regimens. In working with children under communicative restrictions, caregivers can assume a nondirective approach, offering little information but allowing the child to freely discuss feelings, fears, and relationships. When confronted with requests for information, caregivers can help the child identify the people who can address the child's concerns. Caregivers also can serve as quiet advocates for the child's concerns and his or her readiness to assimilate information. Again, it is important to share that approach with parents.

In communicating with children suffering from life-threatening illness, there are two critical points caregivers should recognize. First, it is important to understand what the child is really asking. "Am I going to die?" may not be a request for information but a call for reassurance. Only by asking the child to clarify such questions can the caregivers understand and address underlying concerns.

In one case, for example, a ten-year-old boy asked if his leukemia was fatal. The caregiver began by asking the child what he had heard about the disease. The child talked about a student at his high school, still honored by an annual award presented in her name, who had died of the disease some twenty years earlier. The conversation seemed to indicate that the child wanted reassurance. By honestly discussing the child's anxieties, and by responding to his needs by pointing out that treatment had advanced in the past two decade, the caregiver was able to maintain open communication and hope.

Second, as in any communicative process, each caregiver has to be clear about his or her own role. Perhaps the caregiver may not be the person best suited to answer medical questions. His or her most critical role may be to help the child clarify underlying concerns and questions, identify appropriate resources, and examine the effects of responses on the child's feelings and behaviors.

Truthfulness is not the only thing that can complicate communication with children. Often communication can be complicated by the child's level of cognitive development. Children may not have the vocabulary or conceptual framework necessary to process the information they receive. They may exhibit magical thinking, finding it difficult to separate reality and fantasy. Caregivers can facilitate communication in these situations by patiently providing sufficient time for the child to assimilate information and ask questions. The "report back," a technique in which children recount the information as they understand it, is often an effective way to gain insight in the child's intellectual level and vocabulary, to identify anxieties and feelings complicating the communicative process, and to clarify any misunderstandings. Visual aids appropriate to the age level, such as dolls, models (anatomical models of organs or systems, for example), books, diagrams, and videos can facilitate this communicative process. One physician I know, to help prepare a child for surgery, actually drew the incisions with washable magic marker on the boy's abdomen. This allowed the child two days to get used to the idea of scars and to experiment on what clothes could effectively mask the scaring.

Limits to the child's cognitive development can also impair the task of reviewing life. One of the key tasks in illness is to integrate the illness into one's life. Jewett (1982) suggests that time lines can be an effective way for children to explore the ways that illness has affected their lives. Young children can use different crayon colors to represent periods of life (for example, the child may choose blue for the time before school, green for the time between school and illness, gray for the onset of illness, and so on). Older children can create linear time lines. Such time lines can become the basis for discussion about how they felt and coped during these times and how varied changes in their lives affected them.

Dealing with feelings is another complicated problem for children and adolescents. They may have a difficult time identifying the many emotions they face, and they can find it hard to recognize and assimilate emotions such as anger or guilt. Again, Jewett in her work with bereaved children has developed many techniques that can easily be applied to children with life-threatening illness. Among them are:

1. *Feeling Checks*—This is a simple technique in which the child is asked to tell how much of a given emotion, he/she is experiencing. Younger children may show the emotion by using their hands (close together for little anger, far apart for great anger, and so forth). Older children may demonstrate their level of feeling by selecting a number on a scale. Often the counselor will prepare the child by talking about how some children can have such feelings, thus validating these emotions.

2. *"Five-Five Techniques"*—These refer to a variety of techniques that use five faces (glad, sad, mad, scared, and lonely) (see diagram). These faces may be placed on cards and a number of games may be developed. Children may draw cards explaining when they felt that emotion and how they responded when they felt it. Or they may tell stories about someone who is feeling the emotion expressed on a given face.

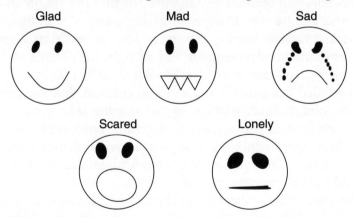

3. *"Show Me"*—Here the caregiver asks the child to "show me how you look sad, or angry, or whatver." This not only gives permission for the feeling but opens discussion of these emotions.

4. *Fables*—In this projective technique the caregiver begins a

"fable" such as "A child wakes up and says 'Oh, I am afraid.'" The child is then asked to complete the fable. Fables can be constructed to uncover any emotion or anxiety.

In addition to these techniques, counselors may wish to use other approaches. Often expressive therapies such as art, play, drama, or music can be useful with children. Jewet, also suggests that counselors should check out family rules about feelings and help children explore their coping by examining how they connect actions with feelings.

Life-threatening illness can often complicate the entire process of a child's or adolescent's development. The process of development is a gradual move toward independence and autonomy. Life-threatening illness can reverse this process, generating greater dependence. Dependence can be complicated by parental overprotectiveness, a common response to a child's illness. Caregivers, children, and parents may need to address these issues, recognizing the child's need for independence and the parents' emotional needs and their deep desire to be involved in care. Often caregivers can help families find mutually agreeable solutions. In one case, for example, parents felt that their adolescent daughter, dying of cancer, was rejecting them. The daughter felt that her fragile independence and dignity was threatened by her parents' response. When they shared their concerns, they were able to reach an agreement on appropriate involvements. It was all right for parents to change her dressing, for that was clearly related to her illness, and she clearly needed her parent's support and comfort. But she preferred to be dressed, bathed, and fed by the nursing staff because if her parents performed those tasks it painfully reinforced her dependency. Such agreements are always tentative and may continually need to be reworked as the child's physical condition changes and the child's development continues.

Adherence issues, especially in the chronic phase, can often be a battleground between parents and children that reflects the struggle between the child's need for independence and autonomy and illness-induced dependency. Often by allowing the child full partnership in treatment; by fully informing the child about the need for adherence; by tailoring the regimen as much as possible to the child's schedule, needs, and life-style; and by soliciting the child's participation in discussions and decisions such conflict can be mitigated. Children and adolescents should be given as many choices as possible during treatment including scheduling times, injection sites, and decisions on who should be present during treatment. Self-help networks, for both parents and children, can also assist both in expressing their feelings and fears, and developing successful coping strategies.

Caregivers should monitor the effects of illness on family life. Because of the great stress of a child's life-threatening illness on the family and the developmental struggle it often creates, there can be deleterious effects upon the family. While earlier observations of extensive marital disruption in families of terminally ill children have not been supported by subsequent research (see Stephenson, 1985) there still may be other negative effects. One study (Hawkins, and Dunkin, 1985) for example, found that in families where children face chronic health conditions there was an increased risk of physical abuse or neglect. Though such situations are rare, monitoring family relationships can sensitize caregivers to the ways that changes in the illness and the child's continued development are affecting family relationships and coping patterns.

It is often worthwhile to explore the family's initial response to the illness. The process of health-seeking is complicated with children, since it can include an additional step in which the child, especially in the older years, has to bring the symptom to the parents' attention and the parents then need to make a decision on seeking help. Exploring this process will often shed light on the family's coping styles; and beliefs about illness. This exploration can also sensitize caregivers to issues that might affect other family members and their responses to the illness. For example, parents who were slow to respond to the child's complaints may face considerable guilt throughout the illness.

This exploration might well include not just family but everyone within the child's circle. Everyone in that circle may be affected by the child's illness. Persons may respond by avoiding the child, or perhaps by overprotecting or overindulging the child. Other parents may prohibit their children from playing with the ill child. The illness may effectively remove the child from arenas for peer interaction, or the child may withdraw and be reluctant to participate in normal activities. Thus it is important to explore the ways that the illness has changed relationships with all those in the child's circle. When caregivers are working within institutions such as hospitals, they may develop support groups for friends and staff.

One important area to explore with school-age children is the response of schools to the illness. I mentioned in Chapter 2 ways that the child's experience of illness may be complicated by school life. Schools can vary in their willingness to accommodate a child's illness and regimen. Some schools will make great efforts to accommodate the child and facilitate adherence to the medical regimen, while others will be resistant to small modicications of routines or regulations. Some schools can be insensitive to a child's threatening illness, perhaps even perceiving education as an unnecessary bother since that child may not survive. Caregivers can assist children and their families in identifying school-based barriers to adherence and help them to develop problem-solving strategies. Some strategies can be as simple as providing the child with privacy for medications or adjusting schedules to accommodate the child's regimen.

Caregivers may also wish to educate schools about symptom control and crisis management. In one case, for example, a nurse and a physician spoke to teachers, a guidance counselor, and a school nurse of an entering high school freshman who had cystic fibrosis. This visit alleviated some fears and allowed the school to identify possible problems that the illness might pose to the child's daily schedule. Once these problems were identified, such as frequent trips to the bathroom, teachers felt more confident that they could handle the child. The guidance counselor appreciated information about the best times to schedule varied courses. Both the school nurse and the guidance counselor also felt relieved at the opportunity to discuss symptoms and their control and to develop crisis management plans. Everyone left the meeting with lists of problems they should watch out for, as well as actions (for example, call the parents; call the ambulance, then call the parents; and so forth) they could take and important emergency numbers. In many cases physicians and other medical personnel can provide information that will alleviate needless fears. In other situations counselors may choose to advocate.

Disclosure concerns can be another school-related issue for both children and parents. Parents may wish to clarify with principals just who would have access to sensitive information. Caregivers may need to help children and parents in clarifying and exploring their concerns. Parents, children, and school staff may also want to develop and periodically review any necessary restriction or emergency and contingency plans. Teachers will need continuous, appropriate, and educationally related information. This information will need to be updated throughout the course of illness. The child's education will be facilitated when teachers and school nurses are incorporated as part of the caregiving team.

Other school-related problems can also develop, particularly during the chronic phase. It is not unusual that the disruptions cased by the disease, the effects of medication and treatment, and the child's responses to the illness can affect cognitive and social development. Caregivers may need to assess such effects with children and their parents, perhaps assisting them to reevaluate their expectations. One young girl suffering from leukemia was deeply distressed that her grades declined and she was no longer able to participate in volleyball. Sensitive to the latter concern, the coach made her his timekeeper when she was able to take this role. While the school also provided access to tutoring, she had to redefine her expectations, recognizing that the maintenance of health was now her highest priority. However, as I pointed out earlier, there may be times that the schools suggest inappropriate placement, placing the child unnecessarily and unsuitably in special education classes or imposing needless restrictions on the child that may run counter to treatment. For example, one school excused a child from physical education even though the doctor felt no such need and suggested exercise. In such cases caregivers can be very effective advocates.

Working with the Developmentally Disabled

One special population that caregivers may come into contact with more frequently these days is the developmentally disabled. In the past two decades more developmentally disabled persons have survived early childhood and are living a longer life span. They are less likely to be living that life within institutions. During the course of that extended life, developmentally disabled persons will experience illnesses in the manner of their nondisabled peers and will be treated for those illnesses within the same facilities and by the same staff. Yet this is a population that will require special sensitivities and approaches from those who care for them.

It is important to remember that the developmentally disabled are not homogeneous. They share the same differences in terms of background as other groups. Levels of cognitive disability can vary from mild to severe. Living conditions can also vary: some may live independently, others with their families or in group homes, still others in institutions. Levels of social and psychological impairments can also differ, and may not neatly correspond to cognitive impairments. Thus an impaired person's age may not be predictive of developmental level or behavior.

Lavin (1989) describes certain characteristics typical of the develomentally disabled. They often have an external locus of control, lack confidence in their own ability to solve problems, find it difficult to think abstractly, have limited ability to transfer skills from one level to another, and have poor short-term memory skills.

Because of these limitations, developmentally disabled persons may ahve a very difficult time coping with abstract concepts such as "disease," "dying," or "death." Some research has suggested that these concepts may be easier for developmentally disabled persons to master as they age. Chronological age, rather than cognitive level, may be a factor, since it provides a rough index of the developmentally disabled person's level of experience with dying and death. Often these conceptual difficulties may be exacerbated by family and staff if they try to overprotect the developmentally disabled client, effectively disenfranchising the client from any role in the treatment.

In discussing grief counseling with the developmentally disabled, Lavin (1989) makes a number of points that can be applied to counseling the developmentally disabled in any crisis. First, she emphasizes the need for caregivers to be patient and clear with their clients. Comfort and continued reassurance may be particularly important throughout the crisis. Second, Lavin emphasizes that caregivers will have to teach coping skills throughout the crisis. This begins by analyzing what behaviors and skills will be necessary at each phase. Lavin then suggests that a four-step process can facilitate learning:

1. *Preparation*—Here the goal is to prepare the developmentally disabled to be exposed to the experience. Caregivers may wish to begin by talking about the individual's previous experiences with illness. This will provide an opportunity to draw upon these experiences in later times.

2. *Direct Instruction*—The caregiver can teach skills that may be useful to the person, providing constant reassurance and reinforcement. For example, he or she may have to go over circumstances in which the individual should notify an appropriate caregiver about changes in health, carefully explaining the symptoms the person might monitor.

3. *Modeling*—In this approach someone models the expected behavior for the individual. The caregiver may help to interpret the event (for example, "He is going to tell the nurse what's bothering him"). The disabled person can then attempt to copy the behavior with the encouragement and support of the caregiver.

4. *Emotional Support*—Throughout the crisis developmentally disabled individuals may have to be helped to understand and express their emotions. Directive questions such as, "Are you scared?" or "How do you feel when you are scared?", may help such individuals to recognize their emotions. Caregivers may need to provide considerable support throughout the crisis of illness. Nonverbal behaviors such as reassuring touch may provide that needed and welcome presence.

Caregivers may find that counseling developmentally disabled individuals requires considerable flexibility in approach. Depending on the level of disability, the present crisis, and the person's previous experiences, caregivers may have to continually adapt approaches to each person. But these clients still share the same needs as other nondisabled individuals, including the need for autonomy, control, and respect.

Working with the Elderly

Though two-thirds of dying persons in the United States are sixty-five years old or older, comparatively little attention has been paid to their unique concerns and issues. Many health-care workers, like other segments of the population, prefer to work with younger clients, often because they have been influenced by negative stereotypes of the elderly. Thus, the elderly ill may face a double burden, rejected both for being old and for dying. We need much more research targeted on the elderly's special requirements and on improving caregiver services for the elderly.

Three basic understandings are fundamental. First, caregivers must realize that the elderly are not a homogeneous group. They differ, as does any age group, on any number of variables such as ethnicity, culture, class, educational level, coping skills, family, and informal and formal support systems.

Second, caregivers must have a basic understanding of the aging process. This includes an ability to distinguish between changes due to normal aging and those that are pathological and/or illness-related. For example, confusion and disorientation are not part of the normal aging process but rather symptoms of underlying disorders that can be either acute and reversible or chronic and irreversible. Should such symptoms become evident during treatment, the individual should be assessed. In some cases disorientation may be caused by dietary changes, medication, or other facts of a treatment program; in other cases disorientation may be a manifestation of the illness or a sign of another condition. These symptoms should not be readily dismissed as evidence of aging. In fact, any symptom, pain, or discomfort experienced by elderly individuals should be viewed with the same seriousness as a complaint by any younger person.

Third, caregivers must examine their own beliefs and feelings about the aging process and the elderly. Are the elderly being treated with respect? Are their needs for independence and autonomy being considered? Are their a psychological and social needs, including sexual needs, being recognized.

Five issues may complicate the elderly's attempts to cope with life-threatening illness and/or their efforts to engage in the counseling process.

RESISTANCE TO COUNSELING/CAREGIVING. Many elderly persons may be resistant to engaging in the counseling process. The reason may be historical. Elderly persons may not have the same familiarity with counseling services as younger people. In addition, the elderly may associate use of mental health services with stigma. The elderly may be reluctant to engage in an activity that they perceive as challenging their autonomy or privacy. Thus it is important for caregivers to be sensitive to such resistance. Counselors and caregivers should try to present the option of counseling in a manner that both explains and normalizes the counseling process. They should not assume that elderly individuals have a clear image of what counseling entails. They should be open to questions and should respectfully examine the misperceptions and anxieties that the elderly may have about the counseling process. For example, one elderly man diagnosed with cancer was reluctant to have a psychological and social work assessment since he feared that the process would inevitable lead to his institutionalization in a nursing home. Naturally, the elderly person's right to reject participation in counseling, should be respected. In such cases the caregiver should reassure the person that the option remains open. Even if an elderly person does agree to counseling, there may be times within the counseling process when the issue of resistance needs to be addressed.

STEREOTYPES ABOUT AGING MAY INHIBIT HEALTH-SEEKING. A second issue that may arise with the counseling process concerns health-seeking behavior. Successful coping with life-threatening illness entails constant monitoring of one's bodily state. While some elderly individuals may exhibit obsessive hypochondrias, other elderly people may ignore, dismiss or discount symptoms. Elderly individuals are just as likely to be deluded by aging stereotypes as their families and others: often they may dismiss symptoms of mental or physical decline as evidence of the aging process. This tendency can be identified when counselors explore the initial process of health-seeking. Here they may find that an elderly client chose self-medication or delayed seeking medical help for a considerable, perhaps even fatal, interval. Once identified, the danger of such strategies can be explored and elderly individuals can be taught more effective strategies for monitoring and supporting health. In some cases these discussions will uncover feelings of fatalism and resignation. For example, one elderly woman delayed seeking treatment for skin cancer. Questioned as to why she had waited so long, she replied that at age eighty-four something was bound to kill you. In other cases this exploration can unveil feelings of guilt and anger: an older person may feel guilty about delaying treatment or angry about the inability of others to treat their complaints seriously.

SOCIAL SUPPORT MAY BE LIMITED. While the issue of social support is not unique to the elderly, it is more likely to be a problem with the elderly than with other age groups. Elderly clients may well have outlived other family members, or surviving family members—wife or husband, siblings, even children—may be too old themselves to be able to help. Thus it is essential for caregivers to ascertain both the size and nature of any possible support system as well as its ability to provide care. Once the support system is identified, caregivers and elderly individuals can assess barriers to its effective utilization, for example, the client's reluctance to request help. Caregivers can assist elderly individuals in identifying additional sources of support. Local offices of aging may be particularly helpful in assisting with needs assessments as well as with identifying, providing, and monitoring supplementary services. Such exploration can uncover significant information about the client's perceptions and misperceptions concerning social support. One eighty-seven-year-old woman, for example, was intensely angry because she though her only daughter should be providing more help. But the daughter herself was near seventy and taking care of an ailing husband. Lack of support can accentuate feelings of loneliness, complicate adjustment to life-threatening illness, and even limit access to varied programs such as hospice that may require the presence of a family caregiver.

OTHER PHYSICAL AND/OR COGNITIVE IMPAIRMENTS. Elderly persons found with life-threatening illness may suffer other cognitive and physical impairments. While such impairments are not an inherent part of the aging process, they become more common as persons age. Naturally, the presence of such impairments has to be considered when developing regimens and when assisting individuals in meeting the tasks necessitated by life-threatening illness. Moreover, the effects and complications of these other conditions and impairments need to be monitored throughout all the phases of illness.

PROBLEMS OF LIFE REVIEW. Finally, elderly persons may have particular conserns connected with the life-review process. While this process is common to all experiencing a sense of finitude, the elderly may have unique concerns. At this point in their lives they may see the unfolding of events that cause them special pain. One elderly man, for example, was distressed to recognize that none of his grandchildren would carry on the family name. In counseling he was able to redefine his concept of family continuity in ways that provided psychological comfort. In similar ways elderly individuals may be deeply distressed about the plight of their survivors, concerned about the ability of spouses, or even adult children, to function without them. One elderly woman, for example, was deeply concerned about the effect of her death upon her husband who was both physically impaired and showing signs of confusion. Another woman was troubled by the fact that she was leaving a retarded son behind. In both cases contingency planning with a caregiver and other relatives eased anxiety.

Caregivers may experience their special stresses as they deal with elderly clients. Caregivers can be troubled by the loneliness of elderly individuals or the plight of survivors. Problems may arise about the appropriateness of care. Given the age and probable continued suffering of an elderly individual, caregivers may be resistant to any form of extraordinary cure.

A Sensitivity to Self

Giving care to persons who have life-threatening illness can be stressful and emotionally draining. Whenever one cares for someone struggling with life-threatening illness, one risks having to confront the death of the client, a consequent sense of loss, and fears associated with one's own mortality, all of which can be profound stresses. Sensitive caregivers should realize that unless they address their own needs, they may have little left to give to others.

Professionals often find it difficult to realize and admit how the losses others experience can affect oneself. One of the most destructive myths about professionalism is that the mark of the profession is to remain emotionally unattached and uninvolved. In fact, caregivers often forge very close relationships with ill individuals and their families. Naturally, crisis points in an illness will affect caregivers, and deaths can be devastating. Moreover, even though a caregiver may feel an intense sense of loss when a special client dies, that sense of loss may not be recognized and validated by others. Even the caregiver himself or herself may not recognize or admit deep feelings of grief. Such grief is real but effectively disenfranchised because the caregiver recognizes no perceived right to mourn.

Caregivers may experience this sense of loss even before families have recognized the extent of their loss. Kastenbaum (1987) describes the phenomena of "vicarious grief" among the elderly. He points out that elderly persons often experience grief "vicariously" when they hear of the losses of younger persons. Kastenbaum suggests that the elderly person, having experience in grief, may empathize more with the newly bereaved, for the elderly person understands the pain and turmoil the newly bereaved are likely to face. Perhaps caregivers undergo a similar experience. Even in the early and more hopeful periods of an individual's illness, caregivers may have the background and experience to anticipate and grieve vicariously for the pain and difficulty persons are likely to face.

The death of a client may cause a caregiver to confront his or her own mortality. Usually by midlife one develops a true awareness of one's own mortality. The deaths of others, particularly when they are close to our own age, may sharpen that awareness of mortality. One grieves not only the loss of another, but a recognized eventual loss of self.

Caregivers may also find it stressful to cope with the choices that individuals make in the course of their illness. For example, many caregivers are personally offended when clients seek alternative treatments and therapies. Rather than understanding this choice for what it is, the decision to explore any path that offers hope, caregivers may experience it as rejection. In such situations caregivers should accept the client's right to choose, and instead of offering dire predictions or condemning the client's decision, the caretaker should make it clear that the welcome mat will always be out. Even at later points in the illness caregivers can be troubled by individual's choices, particularly by decisions to end treatment. As caregivers confront the disparity between their preferred choices and what the ill individuals actually choose, the caregiver's own sense of stress can increase.

Studies have revealed other factors that can contribute to caregiver stress. For example, children and adolescents with life-threatening illness often create unique stress. Individuals with whom caregivers identify, preexisting family problems that complicate an individual's coping, factors related to the particular illness such as its symptoms or trajectory, and a variety of other factors can affect the caregiver's experience of stress and grief.

The work environment often exacerbates caregiver stress. In fact, for many caregivers work difficulties such as communication problems, inadequate resources and support, or structural and role difficulties add greatly to their stress.

Caregivers need to be sensitive to the effects that working with the seriously ill and the dying have on them. Stress and grief may manifest itself physically in minor and major illness. It may emerge in behaviors evident at home or at work, in sleep disturbances, for example, or in psychological reactions such as depression, guilt, anger, irritability, frustration, anxiety, or a sense of hopelessness. It can affect caregiver's cognitive processes, causing errors in judgment or magical thinking.

Caregivers need to be sensitive to their own feelings, and must develop effective coping strategies. Some of these may be structural. Provision for formal support and sharing, both in a group and in an individual context, can be helpful. Ongoing education can provide caregivers with new insights and techniques that enable them to function better. Work flexibility that allows caregivers opportunity to distance themselves and find periodic respite can minimize stress and facilitate grief. Attending funerals or finding other ways to memorialize significant clients may provide a sense of closure.

I once led a session for social work staff of two different agencies. Staff at both agencies were dealing with foster children who were HIV positive. Often children in their care died. The staff in one agency seemed to be coping noticeably better than the staff in the other agency. A critical factor in this difference was the work environment. In the former agency staff had developed a team approach, with weekly support meetings. In the latter agency staff were expected to function autonomously. In the first agency the director set a tone that was very responsive to the emotional needs of staff. She often suggested that staff should go home after they experienced a death, perhaps taking a day or two off. In the other agency the director was concerned that staff not take unanticipated days off, reminding her social workers that they knew the nature of the job when they accepted it. I asked each worker to write down the average number of hours each worked. It was the same for each agency. The flexability in the first agency did not diminish the amount of work accomplished. It did, however, allow staff space and time to meet their own emotional needs.

While structural modifications may help caregivers deal more effectively with their own feelings and reactions, caregivers also need to examine their own personal coping mechanisms.

Weisman (1979) uses a concept that he calls the "least possible contribution" as a way that caregivers can effectively cope with their own stress and sense of powerlessness. Weisman suggests that if caregivers can do something just a bit extra, for example, bake cookies for a person or bring someone a special tape or book, such simple little acts can later help to assuage feelings of grief and loss. The idea is not to do as little as possible, but to try to do something, however small, that will make a difference to a person's life. Studies (Vaenon, 1987) have identified some other factors that may mitigate stress and facilitate grief. One of the most important factors is that caregivers and counselors should develop effective ways to manage their life-styles. Proper rest, good nutrition, exercise, and opportunities for respite, relaxation, diversion, and renewal are all important aspects of life-style mangement. Informal social support can also be a critical factor, especially when support is not available within a professional or work context.

A personal philosophy that both allows one a perspective on the suffering and unfairness evident in life-threatening illness and that defines a professional role in ways that permit a sense of competency and control may also assist coping. In my training of clergy and chaplains, for example, I often talk of a "theology of the unknown" and a "ministry of presence." By the former I mean that clergy have to accept that they cannot explain every act: illness and death are mysteries beyond comprehension. The ministry of presence refers to a role in which clergy and chaplains define themselves as supportive presences, providing comfort and contact rather than resolution. Caregivers have to explore and develop their own philosophies and perspectives on roles that provide them with succor in grief and stress.

Caregivers have a unique role to play in an individual's struggle with life-threatening illness. That role might be compared to a candle. A candle can help illuminate an experience, provide a path in the darkness, and give courage to explore. Caregivers, at their best, can provide that light. That light can accompany individuals as they negotiate a sometimes treacherous and scary path. The journey still be dark, but the light can make it less terrifying.

Conclusion

Over the past forty years there has been a revolution in medical care. Many diseases, that were inevitably fatal are now responsive to treatment and can be cured. In some cases these dieases remain life-threatening, but they are no longer inexorably fatal. In other cases modern treatment can secure a considerable time, between the point of diagnosis and the point of death for the ill individual. And in that time, there may be considerable, even realistic, hope that future medical breakthroughs can further delay, if not defeat, death.

A diagnosis of life-threatening illness is not welcome news, but it usually not an immediate death sentence. It portends struggle, but not necessarily defeat. And it will challenge everyone involved—persons struggling with the disease, their families, and their all caregivers.

Individuals and families will find that their lives are changed by the illness. Individuals will need to decide whether to surrender to despair or to begin a hopeful though uncertain struggle. As they begin that struggle, the resources that they muster, the strengths they draw on, both inside and outside of themselves, may surprise and hearten them. Families too will change as they identify and struggle with their own emotions and needs while simultaneously supporting the ill member and one another.

Caregivers will find their lives touched by those struggles as well. The human capacity for attachment never seems to ebb. So caregivers, despite a history of pain, may find themselves once more engaged. And it is important that caregivers remember their own emotions and needs even as they support others.

The revolution in medical care will create new challenges for everyone. Researchers will need to examine the different responses and reactions that individuals, families, and caregivers may have at different phases of illness, as well as the specific problem caused by each disease and the variety of psychological, social, cultural, spiritual, and other variables that influence adaptation. Educators, counselors, and caregivers will need a renewed sensitivity to the significant issues that arise at each point in the illness.

More than two decades ago Elizabeth Kubler-Ross wrote her classic book, *On Death and Dying*. Her goal then was to sensitize the public and especially health professionals to the very human needs of the dying person, needs that were often lost even as the technological aspects of care so greatly imporved. Further advances both in medical care and our understandings of the needs and reactions of persons with life-threatening illness may suggest more complex models than Kubler-Ross presented. But her goal then still remains relevent today: to humanize care, and to provide comfort and support in the face of life-threatening illness, death, and loss.

Appendix One
Resources

Individuals and families do not have to face the crisis of life-threatening illness alone. There are many resources that can assist families and ill individuals in their struggles. This appendix and the recommendations of physicians and medical staff can be helpful in locating available services. Among the types of services available:

Illness-Based Groups

Many national groups such as the American Cancer Society or local groups offer a wide variety of services to individuals suffering from specific illnesses and also to their families. These services can include self-help groups, counseling, information and referral, as well as other psychological, social, and health-realated services. Services may even include recreational, respite, or camping programs for ill individuals and/or their families. Other organizations offer specialized services to dying children. For example, "Make a Wish" is a national organization dedicated to fulfilling the wishes of dying children. There are over two thousand health-related organizations in the United States. I have listed major ones here in this appendix. Others can be found through hospital and hospices. A complete listing is also available in the *Encyclopedia of Associations* (Gale Research Inc., Detroit, Michigan) which should be available in most libraries.

Major Health-Related Organizations

American Cancer Society
599 Clifton Road
Atlanta, GA 30329
404-320-3333

American Diabetes Association
P.O. Box 25757
1660 Duke Street
Alexandria, VA 22313
703-549-1500

American Heart Association
1320 Greenville Avenue
Dallas, TX 75231
214-373-6300

American Liver Foundation
998 Pompton Avenue
Cedar Grove, NJ 07009
800-223-0179

American Lung Association
1740 Broadway
New York, NY 10019
212-315-8700

Candlelighters Childhood
Cancer Foundation
1901 Pennsylvania Ave. NW,
Suite 1001
Washington, DC 20006
202-659-5136

Cancer Care
1180 Ave. of the Americas
New York, NY 10036
212-221-3300

Cystic Fibrosis Associates
6931 Arlington #200
Bethesda, MD 20814
800-FIGHT CF

Gay Men's Health Crisis
(AIDS)
129 West 20 Street
New York, NY 10011
212-807-6664, 212-337-1950

Make Today Count
1011 1/2 S. Union Street
Alexandria, VA 22314
703-548-9674

National Kidney Foundation
2 Park Avenue
New York, NY 10003

National Multiple Sclerosis
Society
205 East 42 Street
New York, NY 10017
800-624-8236

National Parkinsons
Foundation
1501 NW 9 Avenue
Miami, FL 83136
800-327-4545

National Stroke Association
300 E Hampden Avenue, Suite
240
Englewood, CO 80110-2622
303-762-7922

National Organizations for Granting the Wishes of Terminally Ill Children

Make a Wish Foundation of
America
4601 N 16 St.
Phoeniz, AZ 85016

The Sunshine Foundation

2842 Normandy Drive
Philadelphia, PA 19154

The Dream Factory
P.O. Box 188
Hopkinsville, KY 42240

Counseling Services

Counseling can be very useful for both the individual struggling with illness and all family members. Counselors provide opportunities to explore reactions and feelings, to discuss the ways one is responding to the problems posed by the illness, and to evaluate responses. The Association of Death Education and Counseling (638 Prospect Avenue, Hartford, CT 06105, 203-232-4825) maintains a list of counselors skilled in working with individuals and families as they cope with life-threatening illness. Hospitals, hospices, mental health clinics, and other agencies are other good sources for information and referral.

In selecting counselors, it is important to ask them whether they have special training and expertise in counseling with families and in situations of life-threatening illness. Counselors have their specialties just as physicians do. The issue of rapport is also important. Each person may respond differently to a particular counselor. One will work more effectively if one is comfortable with a counselor. If one does not feel comfortable with a counselor, it is often helpful to discuss this problem with the counselor. If discussion does not help, it may be worthwhile to seek out another counselor.

Since families can be viewed both as a unit or as a group of individuals, it is not unusual for counselors to find it valuable to meet with the family as a whole and with individual members separately. In some cases, counselors may suggest that individual members seek counseling with a different cousenlor. Counselors should explain and explore with client the reasons for their recommendations.

Community-Based Services

Community-based services include:

1. Access services (information and referral)
2. Health care (including home health care)
3. Specialized housing and housing assistance
4. Protective and legal services
5. Transportation services
6. Employment assistance

7. Home assistance (including homemaker and shopping assistance)
8. Personal support (telephone reassurance, friendly visitors, and the like)
9. Nutritional services (including Meals on Wheels)
10. Social services (for example, case coordination, case management, income anf family assistance)
11. Mental health services (for example, family and individual counseling)
12. Specialized services (for example, services for the elderly or for children)

Community-based services may be available from public, private, or volunteer agencies. Many of these services may charge clients using a sliding scale based upon income. Some may be reimbursable under insurance programs. Not all of these services will be available in every geographic area. Each may have their own standards of eligibility. Often local county governments have information and referral services. Often hospitals and offices of aging can provide information and referral, even for clients who are not elderly and their families, since they frequently are aware of services available to the frail, ill, or homebound.

Hospital and Hospice-Based Services

Hospitals and hospices may provide a variety of services beyond services to individuals and their families.

Hospices can be a most valuable resource. Hospices offer what one colleague calls "aggressive comfort care." In other words, they emphasize keeping dying persons comfortable. Hospices offer a variety of services including physical care (often in the home), psychological care, social services, and spiritual support for both dying individuals and their families. Most even provide bereavement services for survivors. A list of hospices in one's local area can be obtained from one's physician or the National Hospice Organization, 1901 North Moore Street, Suite 901, Arrington, VA 22209, (703) 243-5900.

Alternate Institutional Care

In addition to hospitals and hospices, nursing homes and chronic care facilities can provide valued support. Such facilities may also offer a variety of home-care programs such as "nursing home without walls" that can provide remedial and other rehabilitative services at the client's home. They may also provide "day hospitals" and other daycare programs. Some may even provide respite care, a service that provides for the short-term institutionalization of a chronically ill person, providing family caregivers with assistance in family crisis or respite from caregiving responsibilities.

Self-Help Groups

National self-help organizations such as Compassionate Friends and local self-help groups can also provide valued support for individuals and their families in times of life-threatening illness. National groups can provide information on local chapters. Many communities may also have local self-help clearinghouses that will provide assistance in locating local groups. The National Self-help Clearinghouse offers information and referral to self-help groups throughout the United States. Write to:

National Self-Help Clearinghouse
Room 620N
Graduate School and University Center
City University of New York
33 West 42 Street
New York, NY 10036
(212) 643-2944

Other Resources

Churches, synagogues, or other religious organizations may have programs or services such as visitation, counseling, and support groups. Funeral homes may also offer aftercare and grief support programs.

Self-Help Books

Many times self-help books can be a very helpful resource in a crisis. Books can help one to understand the experience, suggest more effective ways to cope, and offer encouragement and hope. The following organizations offer a variety of books about the crisis of life-threatening illness and loss:

Alpha-Omega Venture
1113 Elizabeth Avenue
P.O. Box 735
Marinette, WI 54143-0735
(715) 735-9549

Compassionate Book Service
479 Hannah Branch Road
Burnsville, NC 28714
(704) 675-9687

Your local bookstores also may be able to offer suggestions.

Appendix Two
Examples of Health Care
Proxies and Living Wills

Health Care Proxy

(1) I, _____
hereby appoint _____
 (name, home address, and telephone number)
as my health care agent to make any and all health care decisions
for me, except to the extent that I state otherwise. This proxy shall
take effect when and if I become unable to make my own health
care decisions.

(2) Optional instructions: I direct my proxy to make health care
decisios in accord with my wishes and limitations as stated below,
or as he or she otherwise knows. (Attach additional pages if necessary.)

 _____
 _____

(Unless your agent knows your wishes about artificial nutrition
and hydration [feeding tubes], your agent will not be allowed to
make decisions about artificial nutrition and hydration. See the
preceding instructions for samples of language you could use.)

(3) Name of substitute or fill-in proxy if the person I appoint above is unable, unwilling, or unavailable to act as my health care agent.

_____

(name, home address, and telephone number)

_____

4) Unless I revoke it, this proxy shall remain in effect indefinitely, or until the date or condition stated below. This proxy shall expire (specific date or conditions, if desired):

_____

(5) Signature _____
    Address _____
    Date _____

Statement by Witness (must be eighteen or older)

I declare that the person who signed this document is personally known to me and appears to be of sound mind and acting of his or her own free will. He or she signed (or asked another to sign for him or her) this document in my presence.
Witness 1 _____
Address _____
Witness 2 _____
Address _____

New York Department of Health
Distributed by Concern for Dying
250 West 57th Street, New York, NY 10107
(212) 246-6973

New York Living Will

This Living Will has been prepared to conform to the law in the State of New York, as set forth in the case of *In re Westchester*

County Medical Center, 72 N.Y. 2d 517 (1988). In that case the Court approved the use of a Living Will, stating that the "ideal situation is one in which the patient's wishes were expressed in some form of writing, perhaps a 'living will.' "

I, _____, being of sound mind, make this statement as directive to be followed if I become permanently unable to participate in decisions regarding my medical care. These instructions reflect my firm and settled commitment to decline medical treatment under the circumstances indicated below.

I direct my attending physician to withhold or withdraw treatment that merely prolongs my dying, if I should be in an incurable or irreversible mental or physical condition with no reasonable expectation of recovery.

These instructions apply if I am (a) in terminal condition; (b) permanently unconscious; or (c) if I am minimally conscious but have irreversible brain damage and will never regain the ability to make decisions and express my wishes.

I direct that treatment be limited to measures to keep me comfortable and to relieve pain, including any pain that might occur by withholding or withdrawing treatment.

While I understand that I am not legally required to be specific about future treatments if I am in the condition(s) described above I feel especially strongly about the following forms of treatment.

I do not want cardiac resuscitation.

I do not want mechanical respiration.

I do not want tube feeding.

I do not want antibiotics.

I do want maximum pain relief.

Other directions (insert personal instructions: _____

_____

_____

_____

These directions express my legal right to refuse treatment, under the law of New York. I intend my instructions to be carried out, unless I have rescinded them in a new writing or by clearly indicating that I have changed my mind.

Signed: _____ Date:_____

Witness: _____

Address: _____

_____

Signed: _____Date:_____

Witness: _____

Address: _____

_____

Keep the signed original with your personal papers at home. Give copies of the signed original to your doctor, family, lawyer, and others who might be involved in your care.

(Optional) My Living Will is registered with Concern for Dying (Registry No. _____)

Christian Affirmation of Life*

To my family, friends, physician, lawyer, and clergyman:

I believe that each individual person is created by God our Father in love and that God retains a loving relationship to each person throughout human life and eternity.

I believe that Jesus Christ lived, suffered, and died for me and that his suffering, death, and resurrection prefigured and make possible the death-resurrection process which I now anticipate.

I believe that each person's worth and dignity derives from the relationship of love that God has for each individual person and not from one's usefulness or effectiveness in society.

I believe that God our Father has entrusted to me a shared dominion with him over my earthly existence so that I am bound to use ordinary means to preserve my life but I am free to refuse extraordinary means to prolong my life.

I believe that through death life is not taken away but merely changed, and though, I may experience fear, suffering, and sorrow, by the grace of the Holy Spirit, I hope to accept death as a free human act which enables me to surrender this life and to be united with God for eternity.

Because of my belief:

I request that I be infromed as death approaches so that I may continue to prepare for the full encounter with Chirst through the help of the sacraments and the consolation and prayers of my family and friends.

I request that, if possible, I be consulted concerning the medical procedures which might be used to prolong my life as death approaches. If I can no longer take part in decisions concerning my own future and if there is no reasonable expectation of my recovery from physical and mental disability, I request that no extraordinary means be used to prolong my life.

I request, though I wish to join my suffering to the suffering of Jesus so I may be united fully with him in the act of death-resurrection, that my pain, if unbearable, be alleviated. However, no means should be used with the intention of shortening my life.

I request, because I am a sinner and in need of reconcilitation and because my faith, hope, and love may not overcome all fear and doubt, that my family, friends, and the whole Christian community join me in prayer and mortification as I prepare for the great personal act of dying.

Finally, I request that after my death, my family, my friends, and the who Christian community pray for me, and rejoice with me because of the mercy and love of the Trinity, with whom I hope to be united for all eternity.

Signed_____Date_____

*This document was approved by the Board of Trustees of The Catholic Hospital Association in June. Reprints of the Affirmation will be available soon. For quantity prices contact the Publications Department, The Catholic Hospital Association 1438.

The Christian Living Will

To My Family, Physician, Clergy, Attorney and Medical Facility:
First: I,_____, as a Christian, believe that "Whether we live or whether we die, we are the Lord's"
(Roman's 14.8). If death is certain, so is the faithfulness of God in death as in life. with this high hope to sustain me, I wish to be as responsible in dying as in living.
Second: To this end, I implore all those responsible for my care and knowledgeable of my condition to be completely honest with

me in the event of a terminal illness, so that I may make my own decisions and preparations as much as possible.

Third: If there is no resonable expectation of my recovery and I am no longer able to share decisions concerning my future, I ask that I be allowed to die and not be kept alive indefinitely by artificial means or heroic measures. I ask that drugs be administered to me as needed to relieve terminal suffering even if this may hasten the moment of my death. I am not asking that my life be directly taken, but that my dying be not unreasonably prolonged if my condition is hopeless, my deterioration irreversible, and the maintenance of my life an overwhelming responsibility for my family or an unfair monopoly of medical resources.

Fourth: This request is made thoughtfully while I am in good health and spirits. Even if this document be not binding legally, I beg those who care for me to honor its intent, which is in part to relieve them of some of the burden of this decision. In this way, I take responsibility for my own death and gladly give my life back to God.

Date: _____   Signed: _____

Witness: _____

Reaffirmations:

Date: _____   Signed: _____

_____   _____

Copies given to: _____

_____

_____

Acknowledgments

This work has been influenced and nurtured by many sources. Thus it is both fitting and pleasurable to acknowldge these diverse contributions. The ideas of Avery Weisman and E. Mansel Pattison are clearly evident in these pages. Others too have through their writing or teaching influenced my thinking about life-threatening illness. The ideas of Myra Bluebond-Langner, Herman Feifel, Robert Fulton, Barney Glasser, the late Richard Kalish, Robert Kastenbaum, Nat Kollar, Elizabeth Kubler-Ross, Ilene Lubkin, Victor Marshall, Rudolph Moos, Catherine Sanders, Edwin Shneidman, John Stephenson, Judith Stillion, Anselm Strauss, David Sudnow, Mary Vachon, and Hannelore Wass are all evident in these pages. Charles Corr, Van Pine, and Therese A. Rando have had a special role: not only did their ideas and thoughts influence and stimulate me, but their constant encouragement sustained me. Donald Ford, a friend and physician, was always available to answer any technical or medical questions.

Richard Ellis, Sally Featherstone, and Terry Martin had a very significant role in the development of this manuscript. They read through early drafts, correcting grammar, contributing criticism and ideas, and leaving their mark on these pages. I am proud to acknowledge their considerable contributions. Charles Corr did yeoman service, raising important points at each reincarnation of the manuscript as well as enriching this book by his own work and thoughtful forward. There should be a special place in heaven for him.

My many other colleagues in the Association for Death Education and Counseling (ADEC) and the Foundation of Thanatology also provided constant support. Dana Cable, Roberta Halporn, Jeanne Harper, Jack Kamerman, Clarie Kowalski, Austin Kutscher, Dan Leviton, David Meagher, Jane Nichols, Dennis Ryan, Edie Stark, and Ellen Zinner, to name a few who offered encouragement, criticisms, and opportunities for discussion. Both ADEC and the Foundation of Thanatology presented forums to discuss, to develop, and to learn. Betty Murray and Howard Raether of the National Foundation of Funeral Services and Carol Selinski and Richard Dershimer of the New York State Hospice Association provided similar support and opportunities.

My own college has been supportive in many ways. The gift of sabbatical time provided an extended opportunity for writing. More importantly, I will always appreciated the freedom and opportunity to develop professionally that I have had at the College of New Rochelle. I hope I can provide the same opportunity to my students. I would like to acknowledge the support of President Dorothy Ann Kelly, Senior Vice President Stephen Sweeney, Dean Laura Ellis, and former deans Evelyn Blustein, Edward Miller, and David Paelet. I would also like to recognize the stimulation and support so freely offered by my colleagues in the department, Marguerite Coke and James Magee, as well as the constant collegiality offered by all the faculty.

One of the greatest pleasures in teaching at the College of New Rochelle is the opportunity to teach graduate students, many of whom are caregivers. I have learned much from them in all the courses that I have taught. In the summer of 1990 I began to develop much of the material presented in this book in my "Dying and Death" seminar. The students in that seminar were invaluable contributors. I would like to thank each of them: Mary Barret, Wendy Busch, Yvette Carp, Nancy Eck, Anita Field, Ana Fortoura, Roberta Gavner, Rita Peduto, Wanda Rodrigues, Jean Shea, Carole Stathis, Allie Stokes, and Veronica Whipple.

This book would not have been possible without the secretarial and technical help so generously provided by Heidi O. Caban, Denise Hughes, Vera Mezzaucella, Lorin Peritz, Robin Pierce, and Sally Pure. My research assistant, Anita Field, assisted with editing and research. Our department secretary, Rosemary Strobel, deserves special acknowledgment: without her cheerful efficiency, I would never have had the time and serenity to accomplish anything at all. And I have to acknowledge the help, encouragement, and infinite patience of my editor, Margaret Zusky, and her staff at Lexington Books.

I also need to acknowledge my family and friends, and especially my son, Michael. Their gifts included nurturing, patience, encouragement, and respite. And finally, I need to acknowledge all those people who in their own struggle with life-threatening illness and grief taught me much about dying and living.

References

Adams, David, and Eleanor Deveau (1987)."When a Brother or Sister Is Dying of Cancer: The Vulnerability of the Adolescent Sibling." *Death Studies*, 11, 279–295.

Alberts, Michael S., John Lyons, and Richard Anderson(1988). "Relations of Coping Style and Illness Variables in Ulcerative Colitis." *Psychological Reports*, 62, 71–79.

Anderson, Barbara, and Fredric Wolf (1986)."Chronic Physical Illness and Sexual Behavior." *Psychological Issues*, 54, 168–175.

Aries, Phillippe (1987). *The Hour of Our Death*. New York: Knopf.

Atchley, Robert (1991). *Social Forces and Aging*. (6th ed.) New York: Wiley.

Bard, Morton (1970). "The Price of Survival for Cancer Victims." In A. Strauss (ed.), *Where Medicine Fails*, 99–110. Chicago: Aldine.

Bass, David, Karen Bowman, and Linda Noelker (1991). "The Influence of Caregiving and Bereavement Support on Adjusting to an Older Relative's Death." *Gerontologist*, 31, 32–42.

Becker, Ernest (1963). *The Denial of Death*. New York: Free Press.

Bennett, M. I., and M. S. Bennett (1984). "The Uses of Hopelessness." *American Journal of Psychiatry*, 141, 559–562.

Beilin, Robert (1981). "Social Functions of Denial of Death." *Omega*, 12, 25–35.

Bernardo, Felix (1985). "Social Networks and Life Preservation." *Death Studies*, 8–9, 37–50.

Bloom, S. W. (1965). *The Doctor and His Patient*. New York: Free Press.

Bluebond-Langner, Myra (1978). *The Private Worlds of Dying Children*. Princeton, N. J.: Princeton University Press.

(1987). "Worlds of Dying Children and Their Well Siblings." *Death Studies*, 11, 279–295.

Buckingham, Stephen (1987). "The HIV Antibody Test: Psychosocial Issues." *Social Casework*, 68, 387–393.

Buhrich, N. (1986). "Psychiatric Aspects of AIDS and Related Conditions." *Mental Health in Australia*, 1, 5–7.

Burr, Carolyn Keith (1985). "Impact on the Family of a Chronically Ill Child." In N. Hobbs and James Perrin (eds.), *Issues in the Care of Children with Chronic Illness*, San Francisco: Jossey-Bass.

Burton, Linda (1974). "The Family Coping with a Heavy Treatment Regime." In Burton (ed.), *Care of the Child Facing Death*, 74–86. London: Routledge and Kegan Paul.

Butler, Robert (1963). "The Life Review: An Interpretation of Reminiscence in the Aged." *Psychiatry,* 26, 65–76.

———(1975). *Why Survive? Being Old in America.* New York: Harper and Row.

Carlson, Gregory, and Thomas McCledlan (1987). "The Voluntary Acceptance of HIV-Antibody Screening and Intravenous Drug Users." *Public Health Reports,* 102, 391–394.

Capuzzi, Dave, Douglas Grass, and Susan Friel (1990). "Group Work with Elders." *Generations,* 14, 43–48.

Cassileth, Barrie R., Edward J. Lusk David Miller, Lorraine Brown, and Clifford Miller (1985). "Psychosocial Correlates of Survival in Advanced Malignant Disease?" *New England Journal of Medicine,* 312, 1551–1555.

Cauhill, Rita (1976). *The Dying Patient: A Supportive Approach.* Boston: Little, Brown.

Chandler, Kenneth (1965). "Three Processes of Dying and Their Behavioral Effects." *Journal of Consulting Psychology,* 29, 296–301.

Coe, Rodney (1970). *Sociology of Medicine.* New York: McGraw-Hill.

Cohen, Sanford (1988). "Voodoo Death: The Stress Response and AIDS." In T. Peter Bridge, A. Mirsky, and F. Goodwin (eds.), *Psychological, Neuropsychiatric, and Substance Abuse: Aspects of AIDS,* 95–109. New York: Raven Press.

Coolidge, F. and C. Fish (1983)."Dreams of the Dying." *Omega,* 14, 1–8.

Corr, Charles (1991). "A Task-Based Approach to Coping with Death." Presentation to the Association for Death Education and Counseling, Duluth, Minn., April.

Cousins, Norman (1979). *Anatomy of an Illness.* New York: Norton.

Cummings, E., and W. Henry (1961). *Growing Old: The Process of Disengagement.* New York: Basic Books.

Cytryn, Leon, Peter Van Moore, and Mary Robinson (1973). "Psychological Adjustment of Children with Cystic Fibrosis." In G. J. Anthony and C. Koupernik (eds.), *The Child in His Family: The Impact of Disease and Death,* New York: Wiley and Son.

Dalton, Harlon (1989). "AIDS in Blackface." *Daedalus,* 118, 205–227.

Davis, Fred (1972). *Illness, Interaction and the Self.* Belmont, Calif: Wadsworth.

Deasy-Spinetta, Patricia (1981). "The School and the Child with Cancer." In John Spinetta and Patricia Deasy-Spinetta (eds.), *Living with Childhood Cancer,* St. Louis, MO., Mosby.

Dillard, John (1983). *Multicultural Counseling.* Chicago: Nelson-Hall.

Dingwall, Robert (1976). *Aspects of Illness.* New York: St. Martins Press.

Doka, Kenneth J. (1982a). "The Social Organization of Care in Two Pediatric Hospitals." *Omega,* 4, 345–354

———(1982). "Staff Interaction with the Dying Child". 231–246. In E. Pacholshi and C. Corr (eds.), *Priorities in Death Education and Counseling,* Va: Forum for Death Education and Counseling.

———(1993). *Death and Spirituality.* Farmingdale, N.J.: Baywood Press.

———(1984). "Expectations of Death, Participation in Funeral Arrangements and Grief Adjustment." *Omega,* 15, 119–130.

———(1986). "Death and the Elderly: A Conceptual Review." In R. Pacholski (ed.), *Researching Death,* Lakewood, Ohio: Forum for Death Education and Counseling.

———(1987). "The Dread Disease." *ADEC Forum,* 11, 4–5.

———(1988). "Seeking Significance" In Harold Dick, D. Price, P. Buschman, A. Kutscher, B. Robinstein and F. Forstenzer (eds.) *Dying and Disabled Children: Dealing with Loss and Grief,* New York: Hayworth Press.

———(1989a). "The Awareness of Mortality in Midlife: Implications for Later Life." *Gerontology Review,* 2, 19–28.

———(1989). *Disenfranchised Grief.* Lexington, Mass.: Lexington Books.

Drotar, D, and M. Bush (1985). "Mental Health Issues and Services." In James Perrin (ed.), *Issues of the Care of Children with Chronic Illness,* San Francisco: Jossey-Bass.

De Arment, Daniel (1975). "Prayer and the Dying Patient: Intimacy without Exposure." In J. D. Bone, A. Kutsche, R. Neale, and R. Reeves, Jr. (eds.), *Death and Ministry,* New York: Seabury Press.

DeSpelder, Lynne Ann, and Albert Lee Strickland (1987). *The Last Dance.* Palo Alto, Calif.: Mayfield.

Easson, William (1970). *The Dying Child: The Management of the Child or Adolescent Who Is Dying.* Springfield, Ill.: Charles Thomas.

———(1988). "The Seriously Ill or Dying Adolescent: Special Needs and Challenges." *Postgraduate Medicine,* 8, 183–189.

Eisenberg, Myron, Lafaye Sutkin, and Mary Jansen (1984). *Chronic Illness and Disability through the Life Span: Effects on Self and Family.* New York: Springer.

Ellis, Jon G., and Lillian Ranger (1989). "Characteristics of Suicidal Individuals: A Review:" *Death Studies,* 13, 485–500.

Epley, Rita, and Charles McCagy (1978). "The Stigma of Dying: Attitudes toward the Terminally Ill." *Omega,* 8, 379–393.

Erikson, Eric (1950). *Childhood and Society.* New York: Norton.

Eson, Morris, and Boris Paul (1980). "Stroke Symptoms and Their Implications." In J. Reiffel, R. DeBellis, C. Mark, A. Kutscher, P. Patterson, and B. Schoenberg (eds.), *Psychological Aspects of Cardiovascular Disease,* 195–200. New York. Columbia University Press.

Featherstone, Sally (1991). *Adherence vs. Compliance.* Unpublished paper, Barnes Hospital, St. Louis.

Ferrara, Anthony (1984). "My Personal Experience with AIDS." *American Psychologist,* 39, 1285–1287.

Friedman, Sanford, Paul Chodoff, John Mason, and David Hamburg (1963). "Behavioral Observations on Parents Anticipating the Death of a Child." *Pediatrics,* 32, 610–625.

Fuller, Ruth (1988). "Lovers of AIDS Victims: A Minority Group Experience." *Death Studies,* 12, 1–7.

Fuller, Ruth, Sally Geis, and Julian Rush (1988). "Lovers of AIDS Victims: Psychosocial Stresses and Counseling Needs." *Death Studies,* 12, 1–7.

————(1989). "Lovers and Significant Others." In K. Doka (ed.), *Disenfranchised Grief,* Lexington, Mass: Lexington Books.

Fulton, Robert (1987). "Unanticipated Grief." In Charles Corr and Richard Pachalski (eds.), *Death: Completion and Discovery,* Lakewood, Ohio: Association for Death Education and Counseling.

Fulton, Robert, and Julie Fulton (1971). "A Psychosocial Aspect of Terminal Care: Anticipatory Grief." *Omega,* 2, 91–100.

Garfield, Charles (1979). "The Dying Patient's Concern with Life after Death." In R. Kastenbaum (ed.), *Life after Death,* 45–60. New York: Springer.

Gear, Elizabeth, and L. Allen Haney (1990). "The Cancer Patient after Diagnosis: Hospitalization and Treatment." In E. Clark, J. Fritz and P. Rieker (eds.), *Clinical Perspectives on Illness and Loss,* New York: Charles Press.

Geis, Sally B., Ruth Fuller, and Julian Ruch (1986). "Lovers of AIDS Victims: Psychosocial Stresses and Counseling Needs." *Death Studies,* 10, 43–53.

George, R. L., and T. S. Cristiani (1981). *Theory, Methods, and Processes of Counseling and Psychotherapy.* Englewood Cliffs, N. J.: Prentice-Hall.

Gerber, Irwin (1974). "Anticipatory Bereavement." In Bernard Schoenberg, Arthur Carr, Austin Kutscher, David Peretz, and Ivan Goldberg (eds.), *Anticipatory Grief,* 26–30. New York: Columbia University Press.

Glaser, Barney, and Anselm Strauss (1965). *Awareness of Dying.* Chicago: Aldine.

————(1968). *Time for Dying.* Chicago: Aldine.

Goffman, Erving (1961). *Asylums.* Garden City, N. Y.: Anchor.

————(1963). *Stigma: Notes on the Management of Spoiled Identity.* Englewood Cliffs, N. J.: Prentice-Hall.

Gonda, Thomas, and John Ruark (1984). *Dying Dignified: The Health Professional's Guide to Care.* Reading, Mass.: Addison-Wesley.

Gordon, Norman, and Bernard Kutner (1965). "Long-Term and Fatal Illness and the Family." *Journal of Health and Human Behavior,* 6, 190–196.

Graham-Pole, John, Hannelore Walss, Sheila Eyberg, Luis Cho, and Stephen Olejnik (1989). "Communicating with Dying Children and Their Sibling: A Retrospective Analysis." *Death Studies* 13, 465–483.

Grant, Duncan, and Mark Arns (1988). "Counseling AIDS Antibody-Positive Clients: Reactions and Treatment." *American Psychologist,* 43, 72–74.

Gray, Ross (1988). "Meaning of Death: Implications for Bereavement Theory." *Death Studies,* 2, 309–318.

Gubrium, J. (1975). *Living and Dying at Murray Manor.* New York: St. Martins Press.

Gullo, Stephen V., Daniel Cherico, and Robert Shadick (1974). "Suggested Stages and Response Styles in Life-Threatening Illness: A Focus on the Cancer

Patient." In Bernard Schoenberg, Arthur Carr, Austin Kutscher, David Peretz, and Ivan Goldberg (eds.), *Anticipatory Grief,* 53–78. New York: Columbia University Press.

Gullo, Stephen, and George Plimpton (1985). "On Understanding and Coping With Death during Childhood." In S. Gullo, P. Patterson, J. Schowalter, M. Tallner, A. Kutsher, and P. Brachman (eds.), *Death and Children: A Guide for Educating Parents and Caregivers.* Dobbs Ferry, N.Y.: Tappen Press.

Gustafson, Elizabeth (1972). "Dying: The Career of the Nursing Home Patient." *Journal of Health and Social Behavior,* 13, 226–235.

Gyulay, Jo-Eileen (1978). *The Dying Child.* New York: McGraw-Hill.

Haley, William, and Jeffrey Dolce (1956). "Assessment and Management of Chronic Pain in the Elderly." T Brink (ed.), *Clinical Gerontology: A Guide to Assessment and Interventions,* 425–455. New York: Hayworth.

⸻ (1986). "Assessment and Management of Chronic Pain in the Elderly." In T. Brink (ed.), *Clinical Gerontology: A Guide to Assessment and Intervention,* New York: Hayworth.

Hamovich, Maurice (1964). *The Parent and the Fatally Ill Child.* Los Angeles: Delmar.

Harowski, Kathy J. (1987). "The Worried Well: Maximizing Coping in the Face of Death." *Journal of Homosexuality,* 14, 299–306.

Hawkins, Wesley, and David Dunkan (1985). "Children's Illnesses as Risk Factors for Child Abuse." *Psychological Reports,* 56, 638.

Heller, D. Brian, and Carol Schneider (1978). "Interpersonal Methods for Coping with Stress: Helping Parents of Dying Children." *Omega,* 8, 319, 331.

Herr, John, and John Weakland (1979). *Counseling Elders and Their Families.* New York: Springer.

Hine, Virginia (1979). "Dying at Home: Can Families Cope?" *Omega,* 10, 175–187.

Hinton, John (1960). *Dying.* Baltimore: Penguin Books.

⸻ (1975). "The Influence of Previous Personality on Reaction to Having Terminal Cancer." *Omega,* 6, 95–111.

Hobbs, Nicholas, James Perrin, and Henry Irays (1985). *Chronically Ill Children and Their Families.* San Francisco: Jossey-Bass.

Hogshead, Howard (1976). "The Art of Delivering Bad News." *Journal of the Florida Medical Association,* 63, 807.

Humphrey, Marion (1986). "Effects of Anticipatory Grief for the Patient, Family Member and Caregiver." In T. Rando (ed.), *Loss and Anticipatory Grief,* Lexington, Mass: Lexington Books.

Jewett, Claudia (1982). *Helping Children Cope with Separation and Loss.* Harvard, Mass.: Harvard Common Press.

Kalish, Richard, and David Reynolds (1980). *Dying, Death Transcending.* Farmingdale, N. Y.: Baywood Press. Kalish, Richard (ed.), (1981). *Death and Ethnicity: A Psychocultural Study*. Farmingdale, N. Y.: Baywood Press. (1985). *Death, Grief, and Caring Relationships*. Monterey, Calif:

Kamerman, Jack B. (1987). "Vicarious Grief: An Intergenerational Phenomenon." *Death Studies*, 11, 447–453.

——(1988). *Death in the Midst of Life: Social and Cultural Influence on Death, Grief and Mourning*. Englewood Cliffs, N. J.: Prentice Hall.

Kastenbaum, Robert (1979). *Between Life and Death*. New York: Springer.

——(1986). *Death, Society and Human Experience*. Columbus, Ohio: Charles G. Merrill.

——(1987). "Vicarious Grief: An Intergenerational Phenomenon." *Death Studies*, 11, 447–453.

King, Stanley (1963). "Some Psychological Factors in Illness." In H. Freeman, S. Levine, and L. Reeder (eds.), *Handbook on Medical Sociology*, 99–121. Englewood Cliffs, N. J.: Prentice-Hall.

Klein, Allen (1989). *The Healing of Humor*. Los Angeles: Jeremy P. Tarcher.

Klenow, Daniel, and George Young (1987). "Changes in Doctor/Patient Communication of a Terminal Prognosis: A Selective Review and Critique." *Death Studies*, 11, 263–277.

Koestenbaum, Peter (1971). "The Vitality of Death." *Omega*, 2, 253–271.

Koocher, Gerald, and John E. O'Malley (1981). *The Damocles Syndrome: Psychological Consequences of Surviving Childhood Cancer*. New York: McGraw-Hill.

Krause, Neal (1991). "Stress and Isolation from Close Ties in Later Life." *Journal of Gerontology: Social Sciences*, 40, 183–194.

Kubler-Ross, Elizabeth (1969). *On Death and Dying*. New York: Macmillan.

LaGreca, Anthony (1985). "The Psychosocial Factors in Surviving Stress." *Death Studies*, 9, 23–36.

Lasagna, Lovis (1970). "The Prognosis of Death." In Oliver Brim, Howard Freeman, Sal Levine, and Norman Scotch (eds.), *The Dying Patient*, 67–82. New York: Russell Sage.

Lavin, Claire (1989). "The Developmentally Disabled." In K. Doka (ed.), *Disenfranchised Grief*, Lexington, Mass.: Lexington Books.

Lazarus, Richard (1981). "The Costs and Benefits of Denial." In John Spinetta and Patricia Deasy-Spinetta (eds.), *Living with Childhood Cancer*, St. Louis: Mosby.

Lederer, Henry (1958). "How the Sick View Their World." In G. G. Jaco (ed.), *Patients, Physicians and Illness*, 247–256. New York: Free Press.

Leong, Frederick (1986). "Counseling and Psychotherapy with Asian-Americans: Review of the Literature." *Journal of Counseling Psychology*, 33, 196–206.

Le Shan, Lawrence (1952). "The Safety Prone: An Approach to the Accident-Free Person." *Psychiatry*, 15, 465–469.

——(1969). "Psychotherapy and the Dying Patient." In L. Pearson (ed.), *Death and Dying: Current Issues in the Treatment of the Dying Person*, Cleveland, Ohio: Case Western Reserve University Press.

————(1969). "Psychotherapy and the Dying Patient." In L. Pearson (ed.), *Death and Dying: Current Issues in the Treatment of the Dying Person,* 28–48. Cleveland, Ohio: Case Western Reserve University Press.

Lester, C., and L. Saxxon (1988). "AIDS in the Black Community: The Plague, the Politics, the People." *Death Studies,* 12, 562–571.

Levy, M. H. (1988). "Pain Control Research in the Terminally Ill." *Omega,* 18, 265

Lewis, Oscar (1965). LaVida: A Puerto Rican Family in the Culture of Poverty— San Juan and New York. New York: Random House.

Lieberman, M. (1968). "Psychological Correlates of Impending Death: Some Preliminary Observations." In B. Neugarten (ed.), Middle Age and Aging, Chicago. Aldine.

Lifton, R. J., and G. Olsen (1974). Living and Dying. New York: Bantam Books.

Lipe-Goodson, Pamela and Barbara Goebel (1987). "Perception of Age and Death in Mentally Retarded Adults." Mental Retardation, 21, 68–75.

Lofland, Lyn (1978). The Craft of Dying. Beverly Hills, Calif.: Sage.

Lopez, D., and G. Getzel (1984). "Helping Gay AIDS Patients in Crisis." Social Casework, 65, 387–394.

Lubkin, Ilene (1981). Chronic Illness: Impact and Interventions. Boston: Jones and Bartlett.

Lyter, David, Ronald Valdisern, Lawrence Kingsley, William Amoroso, and Charles Rinaldo (1987). "The HIV Antibody Test: Why Gay and Bisexual Men Want or Do Not Want to Know Their Results." Public Health Reports, 102, 468–479.

MacLachlan, John (1958). "Cultural Factors in Health and Disease." In Patients, Physicians and Illness, (4–105. New York: Free Press.

Magee, James (1988). A Professionals Guide to Older Adults Life Review: Releasing the Peace Within. Lexington, Mass.: Lexington Books.

Mages, N. L., and G. A. Mendelsohn (1979). "Effects on Patient's Lives: A Personological Approach." In G. Stone, F. Cohen, and N. Adler (eds.), Health Psychology: A Handbook, 255–284. San Francisco: Jossey-Bass.

Marshall, Victor (1980). Last Chapters: A Sociology of Aging and Dying. Monterey, Calif.: Brooks/Cole.

Martocchio, Benita (1982). Living While Dying.Bowid, Md.: Robert J. Brady.

Mays, Vickie, and Susan Cocron (1987). "Acquired Immunity Deficiency Syndrome and Black Americans: Special Psychosocial Issues." Public Health Reports, 102, 224–231.

McClowry, S., G. Davies, K. May, E. Kwenkamp, and I. M. Martinson (1987). "The Empty Space Phenomenon: The Process of Grief in the Bereaved Family." Death Studies, 11, 301–374.

McCown, Darlene, and Clara Pratt (1985). "Impact of Sibling Death on Children's Behavior." Death Studies, 9, 323–335.

Mearing, Judith (1985). "Cognitive Development of Chronically Ill Children." In N. Hubbs and J. Perrin (eds.), Issues in the Care of Children with Chronic Illness, 672–697. San Francisco: Jossey-Bass.

Mechanic, David (1968). Medical Sociology: A Selective View. New York: Free Press.

———(1980). "The Experience and Reporting of Common Physical Complaints." Journal of Health and Social Behavior, 21, 146–155.

Meges, N. L., and G. A. Mendelson (1979). "Effects on Patient Lives: A Personological Approach." In G. Stone, F. Cohen, and N. Adler (eds.), Health Psychology: A Handbook, San Francisco: Jossey-Bass.

Meyers, A., E. Kirk Master, C. Jorgensort, and M. Mucatel (1983). "Integrated Care for the Terminally Ill: Variations in the Utilization of Formal Services." Gerontologist, 23, 71–74.

Miles, Margaret, and Alice Demi (1984). "Toward the Development of a Theory of Bereavement Guilt: Sources of Guilt in Bereaved Parents." Omega, 14, 299–314.

Mishler, Elliot (1981). "The Social Construction of Illness." In E. Mishler, L. Amarasingham, S. Hauser, R. Liem, S. Osherson, and N. Waxler (eds.), Social Contexts of Health, Illness and Patient Care, 141–168. Cambridge: Cambridge University Press.

Moody, Raymond (1975). Life after Life. New York: Bantam Books.

Moos, Rudolf (ed.) (1977). Coping with Physical Illness. New York: Plenum Press.

(1984). Coping with Physical Illness 2: New Perspectives. New York: Plenum Press.

Moos, R. H., V. D. Tsu (1977). "The Crisis of Physical Illness: An Overview." In R. Moos (ed.), Coping with Physical Illness, New York: Plenum Press.

Morrissey, James (1963). "A Note on Interviews with Children Facing Imminent Death." Social Casework, 44, 343–345.

Nathan, Laura (1990). "Coping with Uncertainty: Family Members' Adaptations during Cancer Remission." In E. Clark, J. Fritz, and P. Reaker (eds.) Clinical Perspectives on Illness and Loss, New York: Charles Press.

Nimocks, M., L. Webb, and J. R. Connell (1987). "Communication and the Terminally Ill: A Theoretical Model." Death Studies, 11, 323–344.

Noyes, Russell, and John Clancy (1977). "The Dying Role: Its Relevance to Improved Patient Care." Psychiatry, 40, 42–47.

O'Connor, Patrice (1993). "A Clinical Paradigm for Exploring Spiritual Concerns." In K. Doka (ed.), Death and Spirituality, Farmingdale, N. Y.: Baywood Press.

Ostrow, David (1988). "Models for Understanding the Psychiatric Consequences of AIDS." In T. Bridge, A. Mirsky, and F. Goodwin (eds.), Psychological, Neuro-psychiatric and Substance Abuse Aspects of AIDS, New York: Raven Press.

Pattison, E. Mansell (1969). "Help in the Dying Process." Voices, 5, 6–14.

(1978). "The Living-Dying Process." In C. Garfield (ed.), Psychological Care of the Dying Patient, 163–168. New York: McGraw-Hill.

Peterson, David, Pamela Wendt (1990). "Employment in the Field of Aging: A Survey of Professionals in Four Fields." Gerontologist, 30, 679–684.

Phillips, David (1969). Dying as a Form of Social Behavior. Paper delivered at the Annual Meeting of the American Sociological Association, San Francisco, Ca. August.

Pickrel, Jeanette (1989). "Tell Me Your Story: Using Life Review in Counseling the Terminally Ill." Death Studies, 13, 127–135.

Preston, Ronald (1979). The Dilemmas of Care. New York: Elsivier.

Price, Kathy (1988). "Empowering Preadolescent and Adolescent Leukemia Patients." Social Work, 33, 275–276.

Rando, Therese A. (1983). "An Investigation of Grief and Adaptation in Parents Whose Children Have Died from Cancer." Journal of Pediatric Psychology, 8, 3–20.

———(1984). Grief, Dying and Death: Clinical Interventions for Caregivers. Champaign Ill.: Research Press.

———(1986). Loss and Anticipatory Grief. Lexington, Mass: Lexington Books.

Range, L., and S. Martin (1990). "How Knowledge of Extenuating Circumstances Influences Community Reactions toward Suicide Victims and Their Bereaved Families." Omega, 21, 191–198.

Roback, Howard (ed.) (1984). Helping Patients and Their Families Cope with Medical Problems. San Francisco: Jossey-Bass.

Roberts, Maida (1988). Imminent Death as Crisis. Paper presented to the Annual Conference of the Association for Death Education and Counseling, Orlando, Fla., April.

Rose, Natalie (1978). "Toward a Social Theory of Dying." Omega, 9, 49–55.

Rosen, Elliot (1989). "Hospice Work with AIDS-Related Disenfranchised Grief." In K. Doka (ed.), Disenfranchised Grief, 301–312. Lexington, Mass.: Lexington Books.

———(1991). Families Facing Death. Family Dynamics of Terminal Illness. Lexington, Mass: Lexington Books.

Rosenbaum, Ernest. (1978). "Oncology/Hematology and Psychological Support of the Cancer Patient." In C. Garfield (ed.), Psychosocial Care of the Dying Patient, 169–189. New York: McGraw-Hill.

Rosenstock, I. M. (1959). "Why People Fail to Seek Poliomyelitis Vaccination." Public Health Reports, 74, 98–103.

Rothenberg, Michael B. (1974). "Problems Posed for Staff who Care for the Child." In L. Burton (ed.), Care of the Child Facing Death, Boston: Routledge and Keegan Paul.

Rush, B. F. (1974). "A Surgical Oncologist's Observation." In B. Schoenberg, A. Carr, A. Kutscher, D. Peretz, and I. Goldberg (Eds.) Anticipatory Grief, 97–106. New York: Columbia University Press.

Ruskin, H. D. (1980). "Care of the Patient with Coronary Heart Disease." In J. Reiffel, R. DeBellis, L. Mark, A. Kutscher, P. Patterson, and B. Schoenberg (eds.), Psychosocial Aspects of Cardiovascular Disease: The Life-Threatened Patient, Family and Staff, 4–14. New York: Columbia University Press.

Ryan, Dennis (1993). "Death: Eastern Perspectives." In K. Doka (ed.), Death and Spirituality, Farmingdale, N. Y.: Baywood Press.

Rybarczyk, Bruce, and Stephen Averback (1990). "Reminiscence Interviews as Stress Management Intervention for Older Patients Undergoing Surgery." Gerontologist, 30, 522–528.

Sanders, Catherine (1983). "Effects of Sudden vs. Chronic Illness Death on Bereavement Outcome." Omega, 13, 227–241.

————(1989). Grief: The Mourning After. New York: Wiley and Sons.

Sanders, Glenn, and Jerry Suls (1982). The Social Psychology of Health and Illness. Hillsdale, N. J.: Erlbaum.

Sankar, Andrea (1991). "Ritual and Dying: A Cultural Analysis of Social Support for Caregivers." Gerontologist, 31, 43–50.

Saunders, Judith M., and S. M. Valente (1987). "Suicide Risk among Gay Men and Lesbians: A Review." Death Studies, 11, 1–23.

Schultz, Richard, and David Aderman (1974). "Clinical Research and the Stages of Dying." Omega, 5, 137–143.

Shneidman, Edwin (1973). Death of Man. Baltimore: Penguin.

————(1978). "Some Aspects of Psychotherapy with Dying Persons." In C. Garfield (ed.), Psychosocial Care of the Dying Patient, New York: McGraw-Hill.

Shneidman, Edwin, and Norman Farbarow (1957). Clues to Suicide. New York: McGraw-Hill.

Siblinga, M. S., C. J. Friedman, and N. N. Huang (1973). "The Family of the Cystic Fibrosis Patient." In P. Patterson, C. Denning, and A. Kutscher (eds.), Psychosocial Aspects of Cystic Fibrosis: A Model for Chronic Lung Disease, 13–18. New York: Foundation of Thanatology.

Siegel, Bernie S. (1986). Love, Medicine and Miracles. New York: Harper and Row.

Skelton, J. A., James Pennebaker (1982). "The Psychology of Physical Symptoms and Sensations." In Glenn Sanders and Jerry Suls (eds.), The Social Psychology of Health and Illness, 99–128. Hillsdale, N. J.: Erlbaum.

Slaby, A., and A. S. Glicksman (1985). Adapting to Life-Threatening Illness. New York: Praeger.

Smith, Walter (1985). Dying in the Human Life Cycle: Psychological Biomedical and Social Perspectives. New York: Holt, Rinehard and Winston.

Smith, William David (1978)."Black Perspectives on Counseling." In Garry Walz and Libby Benjamin (eds.), Transcultural Counseling: Needs Programs and Techniques. New York: Human Sciences Press.

Sontag, Susan (1978). Illness as Metaphor. New York: McGraw-Hill.

————(1988). AIDS and Its Metaphors. New York: Farrar, Straus and Giroux.

Spector, Rachel (1985). Cultural Diversity in Health and Illness. Norwalk, Conn.: Appleton-Century-Crofts.

Spiegel, David, Helena Kraemer, Joan Bloom, and Ellen Gortheil (1989). "Effects of Psychosocial Treatment of Survival of Patients with Metastic Breast Cancer." lancet, 10 (14), 888–891.

Spinetta, John, and Patricia Deasy-Spinetta (1981). Living with Childhood Cancer. St. Louis: Mosby.

Spinetta, John, Helen McKaren, Robert Fox, and Steven Sparta (1981). "The Kinetic Family Drawing in Childhood Cancer." In Living with Childhood Cancer, John Spinetta and Patricia Deasy-Spinetta (eds.), St. Louis: Mosby.

Stearns, Naomi (1990). "A Question of Survival." Illness, Crisis and Loss,Philadelphia, PA: Coaries Press.

Stein, S., M. W. Linn, and E. M. Stein (1989). "Psychological Correlates of Survival in Nursing Home Patients." Gerontologist, 29, 224–228.

Stephenson, John S. (1985). Death, Grief and Mourning: Individual and Social Realitis. New York: Free Press.

Stillson, Judith (1985). Death and the Sexes. Washington, D.C.: Hemisphere.

Strauss, Anselm (1975). Chronic Illness and the Quality of Life. St. Louis: Mosby.

Strauss, Anselm, and J. Wiet Corbin (1988). Shaping a New Health System. San Francisco: Jossey-Bass.

Stulberg, Ian, and Margaret Smith (1988). "Psychosocial Impact of the AIDS Epidemic on the Lives of Gay Men." Social Work, 33, 277–281.

Sudnow, David (1968). Passing On: The Social Organization of Dying. Englewood Cliffs, N. J.: Prentice-Hall.

Sue, Derald Wingsue (1981). Counseling the Culturally Different. New York: Wiley.

Taylor, Phyllis (1983). The Patients' Pain: Strategies for Caregivers. Presentation to Philadelphia Chapter of the Forum for Death Education and Counseling, January.

Thormen, George (1982). Helping Troubled Families: A Social Work Perspective. Chicago: Aldine.

Twaddle, Andrew, and Richard Hessler (1977). A Sociology of Health. St. Louis: Mosby.

Vachon, Mary (1987). Occupational Stress in the Care of the Critically Ill, the Dying, and the Bereaved. New York: Hemisphere.

Verwoerdt, A. (1966). Communication with the Fatally Ill Child. Springfield, Ill.: Charles E. Thomas.

Viney, Linda, and Mary Westbrook (1986). "Is There a Pattern of Psychological Reactions to Chronic Illness Which Is Associated with Death?" Omega, 17, 169–181.

Wadesworth, John S., and Dennis Harper (1985). "Grief and Bereavement in Mental Retardation: A Need for New Understanding." Death Studies, 15, 281–292.

Wahl, Charles (1973). "Psychological Treatment of the Dying Patient." In R. Davis Fed. Dealing with Death, 9–33. Los Angeles: Andrus Gerontological Center.

Walsh, Patricia, and Anthony Walsh (1987). "Self Esteem and Disease Adaptation among Multiple Sclerosis Patients." Journal of Social Psychology, 127, 669–671.

Walum, Laurel (1977). The Dynamics of Sex and Gender: A Sociological Perspective. Chicago: Rand McNally.

Watson, W., and P. J. Maxwell (1977). Human Aging and Dying: A Study in Sociocultural Gerontology. New York: St. Martins Press.

Waxler, Nancy (1984). "Learning to Be a Leper: A Case Study in the Social Construction of Illness." In Elliot Mishler, Lorne Amarsingham, Ramsey Liam, Samuel Sherson, and Nancy Wexler (eds.), Social Contexts of Health, Illness, an Patient Care, 169–194. Cambridge: Cambridge University Press.

Weisman, Avery (1972). On Dying and Denying: A Psychiatric Study of Terminality. New York: Behavioral Publications.

———(1980). "Thanatology." In O. Kaplan (ed.), Comprehensive Textbook of Psychiatry. Baltimore: Williams and Williams.

———(1986). The Coping Capacity: On the Nature of Being Mortal. New York: Human Sciences Press.

Weisman, Avery, and J. William Worden (1975). "Psychosocial Analysis of Cancer Deaths." Omega, 6, 61–75.

———(1979). Coping with Cancer. New York: McGraw Hill.

Wendler, Klaus (1987). "Ministry to Patients with Acquired Immune Deficiency Syndrome: A Spiritual Challenge. Journal of Pastoral Care, 41, 4–16.

Williams, Holly Ann (1985). Perceived Needs and Support Systems of Single Parents of Children Diagnosed with a Life-Threatening Disease. Paper presented to the Association of Death Education and Counseling. Philadelphia, April.

Wilson, Robert (1970). The Sociology of Health: An Introduction. New York: Random House.

Winiarski, Mark (1991). AIDS-Related Psychotherapy. New York: Pergamon Press.

Witte, Kim (1991). "The Role of Culture in Health and Disease." In L. Samour and R. Porter (eds.), Intercultural Communication (6th ed.), Belmont, Calif: Wadsworth.

Worden, J. William (1972). "On Researching Death." Pastoral Psychology, 23, 5–8.

———(1982). Grief Counseling and Grief Therapy. New York: Springer.

Wolinsky, F. (1980). The Sociology of Health: Principles, Professions and Issues. Boston: Little, Brown.

Wortman, Camille, and Jack Brehm (1975). "Responses to Uncontrollable Outcomes: An Integration of Resistance Theory and the Learned Helplessness Model." In Leonard Berkowitz (ed.), Advances in Experimental Social Psychology, 217–236. New York: Academic Press.

Zborowski, M. (1952). "Cultural Components in Responses to Pain." Journal of Social Issues, 8, 16–30.

Index